Mastering Scientific and Medical Writing

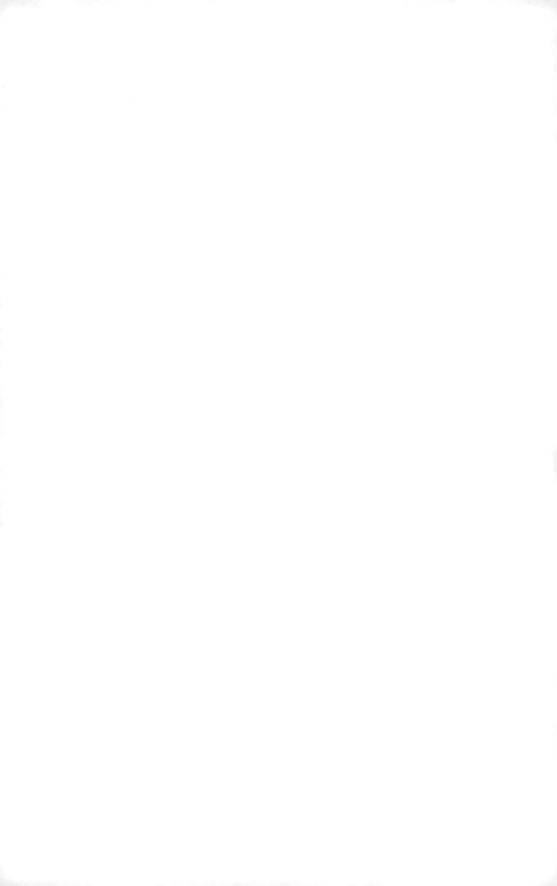

Silvia M. Rogers

Mastering Scientific and Medical Writing

A Self-Help Guide

Second Edition

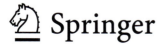

Silvia M. Rogers
MEDIWRITE GmbH
Basel
Switzerland

ISBN 978-3-642-39445-4   ISBN 978-3-642-39446-1   (eBook)
DOI 10.1007/978-3-642-39446-1
Springer Heidelberg New York Dordrecht London

Library of Congress Control Number: 2013955578

© Springer-Verlag Berlin Heidelberg 2014
This work is subject to copyright. All rights are reserved by the Publisher, whether the whole or part of the material is concerned, specifically the rights of translation, reprinting, reuse of illustrations, recitation, broadcasting, reproduction on microfilms or in any other physical way, and transmission or information storage and retrieval, electronic adaptation, computer software, or by similar or dissimilar methodology now known or hereafter developed. Exempted from this legal reservation are brief excerpts in connection with reviews or scholarly analysis or material supplied specifically for the purpose of being entered and executed on a computer system, for exclusive use by the purchaser of the work. Duplication of this publication or parts thereof is permitted only under the provisions of the Copyright Law of the Publisher's location, in its current version, and permission for use must always be obtained from Springer. Permissions for use may be obtained through RightsLink at the Copyright Clearance Center. Violations are liable to prosecution under the respective Copyright Law.
The use of general descriptive names, registered names, trademarks, service marks, etc. in this publication does not imply, even in the absence of a specific statement, that such names are exempt from the relevant protective laws and regulations and therefore free for general use.
While the advice and information in this book are believed to be true and accurate at the date of publication, neither the authors nor the editors nor the publisher can accept any legal responsibility for any errors or omissions that may be made. The publisher makes no warranty, express or implied, with respect to the material contained herein.

Printed on acid-free paper

Springer is part of Springer Science+Business Media (www.springer.com)

Preface

> *"If any man wish to write in a clear style,*
> *let him first be clear in his thoughts."*
>
> Johann Wolfgang von Goethe

You may ask why anyone would want to write yet another book about scientific writing. There are many books on the subject, some more useful than others, and the abundance of literature on this topic may confuse rather than guide.

I felt that this book was necessary for several reasons. During the past years, I have learnt much about the needs of scientific communicators, both through my personal experience as a pharmacologist and, later, through teaching scientific writing at universities, pharmaceutical companies, and other institutions. In today's busy world, guidance on scientific writing must be focused and to the point. Our constraints no longer permit the time-consuming debate about the "correct" word or formulation. Moreover, the speed by which we produce a manuscript has become increasingly important, be it in academia or the pharmaceutical industry. Scientists often find it difficult to accept that their professional success essentially depends on their skill and efficiency to communicate their research results. Without any doubt, the rapid exchange of pertinent information is critical to scientific advancement and should therefore be regarded with due respect.

A second, perhaps even more important reason for writing this book is my personal concern for everyone challenged to write high-quality texts in a language that is not his or her native tongue. As a Swiss-Anglo hybrid (as I like to call myself), I sympathize with their special circumstances and wish to make a contribution to overcoming linguistic dilemmas.

In short, this book deals with clear, unambiguous language within and across the biological and medical sciences. Unlike textbooks on English grammar that analyze and prescribe the use of the language in its various forms, this book tells you how to apply your existing language skills to scientific communication. If you do not only want to write but want to write *well*, this book is for you.

I have used a number of symbols to draw your attention to definitions or rules, examples of the principles stated, or exercises on the subject. This table shows the symbols:

SYMBOL	… AND WHAT IT MEANS
!	Definition or rule
●	Example
>	Exercise

Basel, Switzerland   Silvia M. Rogers

About the Author

Silvia M. Rogers, BSc hons., PhD, is the founder and owner of MEDIWRITE, a successful small company in Basel, Switzerland. She trained at the University of Liverpool, UK, in the Department of Pharmacology and Therapeutics headed by Professor Sir Alasdair Breckenridge. Before forming MEDIWRITE in 1994, she gained extensive experience in key areas of pharmaceutical research, including project management in a major pharmaceutical company. She is an active member of the American Medical Writers Association (AMWA) and the European Medical Writers Association (EMWA). She lectures on scientific writing at the University of Basel and has provided extensive training in various aspects of medical and scientific writing and presentation. She has written numerous expert reports, regulatory documents, scientific publications, and study reports for clients.

Acknowledgments

First and foremost, my thanks go to my workshop participants and university students of the past 15 years, without whom this book would not have been written. Their active participation, questioning, and challenging of issues during workshops and lectures encouraged me to put into print the most important aspects of scientific writing.

I am most grateful to my colleagues whose input greatly helped to shape the contents of this book. Moreover, I gratefully acknowledge the astuteness and competence of my proofreaders. My special thanks go to Lea Streule, whose meticulous attention to detail was of tremendous help.

Finally, I am indebted to the readers of the first edition of this book. Owing to their interest in scientific communication and their useful comments, this second edition became possible.

Contents

1	**Introduction**...	1
2	**Good Versus Poor Scientific Writing: An Orientation**	3
	2.1	What Is "Good" Scientific Writing?	3
	2.2	The Plain Language Movement.	4
	2.3	The BASO Pyramid of Scientific Writing.	5
		2.3.1 Baseline	6
		2.3.2 Style.	6
		2.3.3 Opinion	6
	2.4	Common Myths and Misconceptions	7
		2.4.1 What Are Myths and Misconceptions?..............	7
		2.4.2 Long and Complicated Sentences	8
		2.4.3 Misusing or Wasting Specific and Generic Terms......	8
		2.4.4 Reluctance to Use First-Person Pronouns Leading to Overuse of Passive Voice.	9
		2.4.5 Tendency to Turn Sharp and Powerful Verbs into Weighty Nouns.............................	9
3	**Words and Units: Orthography and Punctuation**	11
	3.1	Correct Spelling.	11
		3.1.1 Getting Words Right	11
		3.1.2 Using Spell Checkers.	12
	3.2	Consistent Spelling: American English Versus British English.....	12
	3.3	Punctuation	13
		3.3.1 Proper Use of Punctuation Marks	13
		3.3.2 Hyphens and Word Division	13
		3.3.3 Punctuation Marks Indicating Emotion...............	15
		3.3.4 Parentheses and Brackets.........................	15
		3.3.5 Periods in Titles and Academic Degrees.............	16
		3.3.6 Apostrophes in Contractions	17
		3.3.7 Nonbreaking Spaces and Hyphens	17
	3.4	Shortened Word Forms in Scientific Writing	18
		3.4.1 Types of Abbreviations	18
		3.4.2 True Abbreviations	19
		3.4.2.1 Latin Abbreviations	19

		3.4.3	Units of Measurement	19
		3.4.4	Acronyms and Initialisms	21
		3.4.5	Contractions	21
		3.4.6	Suspensions	22
	3.5	Numbers		22
		3.5.1	Expressing Numbers in Scientific Texts	22
		3.5.2	Formats of Numbers	23
		3.5.3	Ranges of Numbers	24
		3.5.4	Percentages	24
	3.6	Capitalization		25
		3.6.1	Use of Capitals in Scientific English	25
		3.6.2	Capitals in Proper Nouns (Names)	25
		3.6.3	Capitals in Titles	26
			3.6.3.1 Capitalizing Hyphenated Compound Words in Titles	26
		3.6.4	Capitals in Designations	27
		3.6.5	Capitals in New-Age Words	27
4	**Forming Sentences: Grammar**			**29**
	4.1	Why Battle with Grammar?		29
	4.2	The Tenses in Scientific Reporting		30
	4.3	Joining Statements		32
		4.3.1	How Can the Joining of Words or Statements Cause Confusion?	32
		4.3.2	Nonparallel Verbs	33
		4.3.3	Nonparallel Modifiers	34
		4.3.4	Nonparallel Prepositional Phrases	35
	4.4	Subject–Verb Agreement		35
		4.4.1	Using the Correct Verb Forms	35
		4.4.2	Special Nouns	37
		4.4.3	Collective Nouns	37
		4.4.4	The Rule of Meaning	38
		4.4.5	Verb Matching with "None" and the "Neither–Nor" Linkage	39
	4.5	Syntax (Order of Words)		40
		4.5.1	Modifying Phrases	40
		4.5.2	Position of Adverbs in Sentences	41
		4.5.3	Position of Prepositions in Sentences	42
	4.6	Dangling Participles (and Other Danglers)		43
		4.6.1	What Are Danglers?	43
		4.6.2	Dangling Participles	43
		4.6.3	Dangling Gerunds	45
	4.7	The Relative Pronouns "Which" and "That"		45
	4.8	Use of "Respectively"		46
	4.9	Plurals of Abstractions and Attributes		47

5	**Putting It Nicely: Style**		49
	5.1	What Is "Style" in the Context of Scientific Writing?	49
	5.2	Active Versus Passive Voice	50
		5.2.1 Why Argue About Active/Passive Voice?	50
		5.2.2 Shifting Emphasis by Choosing the Voice	50
		5.2.3 The Verb "To Be" in Copula Formulations	51
	5.3	Overuse of Prepositions	51
	5.4	Limiting Modifiers and Other Decorative Words	53
		5.4.1 Excessive Adjectives, Adverbs, and Nouns	53
		5.4.2 Modifier Strings	54
	5.5	The "House Style" of Journals	55
	5.6	Company-Internal Conventions of Style and Format	56
6	**Redundancy and Jargon: Focusing on the Essentials**		59
	6.1	Redundancies in Scientific Reporting	59
	6.2	Double Negatives	60
	6.3	Tautology (Repeated and Redundant Words)	60
	6.4	Doubling Prepositions	61
	6.5	Jargonized Writing	62
	6.6	Oxymorons	63
7	**Quoting Published Material: Reference Formats**		65
	7.1	What Can Go Wrong When Quoting Published Material?	65
	7.2	Reference Formats and the Uniform Requirements	66
		7.2.1 What Style Should I Use?	66
		7.2.2 Using Vancouver Style	66
		7.2.3 Reference Manager Tools	69
8	**Ethics of Scientific Writing: Avoiding Discrimination**		71
	8.1	Prejudice and Semantic Labeling	71
	8.2	Sexist Writing and Gender-Biased Expressions	71
		8.2.1 Sex Versus Gender	71
		8.2.2 Gender-Inclusive Language	72
	8.3	Racist Writing	73
	8.4	Ageism	74
9	**Sticking to Your Word: Avoiding Plagiarism**		75
	9.1	What Is Plagiarism?	75
	9.2	Forms of Plagiarism	76
		9.2.1 Plagiarism of Text	76
		9.2.2 Plagiarism of Ideas	77
		9.2.3 Self-Plagiarism	78
	9.3	How to Avoid Plagiarism	79
10	**Structuring Scientific Texts: Getting the "Story" out**		81
	10.1	Determining the Audience	81
	10.2	Adapting the "Story" to the Readers' Needs	82

		10.3	Drafting an Abstract	83
			10.3.1 The Importance of Abstracts	83
			10.3.2 Descriptive Abstracts	84
			10.3.3 Informative Abstracts	84
			10.3.4 Structured Abstracts	84

11 Appendix ... 85
    11.1 Scientific Writing Rules at a Glance ... 85
    11.2 American English Versus British English: Groups of Words Affected by the Different Spelling ... 88
    11.3 The Main Punctuation Marks in Scientific Writing ... 89
    11.4 Awkward Phrases to Avoid ... 91
    11.5 List of Academic Degrees and Honors ... 94

12 Exercises ... 97
    12.1 Exercise 1 | Consistent Spelling ... 97
    12.2 Exercise 2 | Proper Punctuation ... 97
    12.3 Exercise 3 | Using Numbers and Percentages Correctly ... 98
    12.4 Exercise 4 | Using Proper Capitalization ... 99
    12.5 Exercise 5 | Using Tenses in Scientific Reporting ... 99
    12.6 Exercise 6 | Restoring Parallelism ... 100
    12.7 Exercise 7 | Avoiding Verbal Phrase Danglers ... 101
    12.8 Exercise 8 | Using "Respectively" Properly ... 101
    12.9 Exercise 9 | Avoiding Excessive Passive Voice ... 102
    12.10 Exercise 10 | Limiting the Number of Prepositions ... 102
    12.11 Exercise 11 | Using Modifiers in Moderation ... 103
    12.12 Exercise 12 | Avoiding Tautological and Other Redundant Expressions ... 103

13 Solutions to Exercises ... 105
    13.1 Solutions to Exercise 1 ... 105
    13.2 Solutions to Exercise 2 ... 106
    13.3 Solutions to Exercise 3 ... 107
    13.4 Solutions to Exercise 4 ... 107
    13.5 Solutions to Exercise 5 ... 108
    13.6 Solutions to Exercise 6 ... 109
    13.7 Solutions to Exercise 7 ... 110
    13.8 Solutions to Exercise 8 ... 110
    13.9 Solutions to Exercise 9 ... 111
    13.10 Solutions to Exercise 10 ... 112
    13.11 Solutions to Exercise 11 ... 112
    13.12 Solutions to Exercise 12 ... 113

References ... 115

Introduction   1

*"The way we express ourselves
portrays the way we think."*

The main purpose of scientific writing is to record data. Without a written record of our findings, there is no proof that we have done the research, and precious information may be lost. Many experiments may have to be repeated, simply because there is no record of the data. Needless to say, this negligence adversely impacts on the efficiency of sharing scientific knowledge.

One of the main challenges of scientific writing is to pack vast and complex information into clear and well-structured texts. It is a skill that requires not only knowledge of the scientific field but also practice in writing. Uncertainties about the required style and format of scientific papers may delay publication of important new findings.

We must bear in mind that scientific writing differs substantially from literary writing. While literary writing is an art based on principles of personal style, fiction, and originality, *good* scientific writing is a craft that builds on clear communication of scientifically researched facts.

Good scientific writing hinges on the ability to express complicated concepts in clear words, thus pointing out the beauty of science without unnecessary decoration. Although we would all agree that the beauty of science is in the science *itself*, not in the language used to describe it, we have to accept that a confusing account of our findings will not do justice to the science that lies behind it.

What can we, as writers, do to ensure that our scientific message reaches the intended target population?

Good scientific writing is
- *understandable*: Readers should *read* our paper in full, rather than discarding it after a few sentences because the text makes no sense to them. We should also bear in mind that while the international scientific language is English, the native tongue of readers (other scientists, regulators, etc.) may be a language other than English.

- *transparent*: The written report is often the only way for readers to access the research done. Thus, our scientific paper is the only "window" through which readers can view our "laboratory."
- *clear*: Some scientists inadvertently keep their acquired knowledge to themselves rather than share it with the scientific community or their peers. They may write in a vague, complicated, and unstructured manner, using ample ornamentation that distracts the reader. However, good scientific writing should inform rather than confuse the readers.
- *credible*: As scientists, we have to be credible to gain our readers' respect. For instance, if we apply for a research grant, our written proposal must be convincing, both in terms of the concepts and the language used to describe them. Similarly, a paper written in an accurate, compelling, and logical style conveys to the readers that the research described was also done accordingly. The way we express ourselves portrays the way we think.
- *efficient*: By improving our scientific writing skills, we essentially gain time. Poorly written papers may be delayed or even rejected although the science behind them may be of considerable interest. A reputation of being a good and reliable scientific writer will open doors to more publishing and positive feedback.
- *simple*: Text devoid of unnecessary decorative words is more readily understood than complicated, ornamental expositions.

> ! Successful communication in science involves clarity and simplicity, short sentences, transparency, and consistency.

Good Versus Poor Scientific Writing: An Orientation

> "Everything that can be thought at all
> can be thought clearly.
> Everything that can be said
> can be said clearly."
>
> Ludwig Wittgenstein

2.1 What Is "Good" Scientific Writing?

When we declare that a certain text is better than another, we rely on a scale of values, with "good" at one end and "poor" at the other.

But who sets the standards for "good" and "poor" scientific writing? Who is the ultimate judge? Who censors the quality of our scientific texts? While general opinion of what is "correct" may be divided, there are certain bodies or sources that we usually accept as authorities. These include

- dictionaries
- grammarians, linguists, editors, and teachers
- scientific community
- set traditions and accepted trends.

Nevertheless, even experts may disagree among themselves. I have seen groups of learned scientists brooding over a paper, in an attempt to decide whether the paper is well written or not. Opinions often clash, and precious time may be lost because of unnecessary arguments over issues of style that may not affect the clarity of the message.

The ultimate judgment of the quality of our scientific writing efforts lies with the readers themselves. If the learned reader follows our train of thought and understands our message, then the writing has fulfilled its primary purpose.

Nonetheless, we have conventions to follow, guidelines to adhere to, and trends to observe. The changes and trends we have seen over the years could almost be called evolutionary. Many of the rules for good scientific writing valid 10 or 20 years ago have been modified, undone, or even reversed during subsequent years. An example of this phenomenon is the issue of active versus passive writing (see Sect. 5.2). While the passive style of writing used to be the favored voice in the past, it is the active voice that is clearly preferred today.

When evaluating the "power" of a scientific manuscript – your own or some other author's – you may find it helpful to consult the document standards listed in Table 2.1.

Table 2.1 Document Standards

STANDARD	DESCRIPTION
Purpose	The purpose and objectives of the study must be obvious and unambiguous.
Conformity	Text has to conform to given formats and style requirements (see Sect. 5.5, for example).
Accuracy	The wording must be grammatically correct, concise, and precise. All information and data provided must be accurate.
Consistency	Terminology should be consistent and appropriate. Only commonly known abbreviations should be used, and these must be used consistently.
Logic and flow	The manuscript should be a "story" with a clear message based on a logical train of thought.
Context	New findings must be reported and interpreted in the context of findings already published and must be congruent with accepted institutional or regulatory values.
Structure	A logical structure (i.e., headings and subheadings, paragraphs, and data displays) should be chosen. A well-balanced mixture of text and visuals (e.g., figures and tables) should be chosen, in line with the relevant instructions for authors.
Data presentation	High-quality data should be presented clearly, using tables and figures as appropriate. Duplication of data displays must be avoided.

2.2 The Plain Language Movement

In the USA, the plain language movement dates back to the 1970s when the US federal government began encouraging its regulation writers to be less bureaucratic. Meanwhile, many agencies have introduced policies that enforce the use of plain language for academic, legal, and other professional texts. In 2010, the use of plain English became a federal requirement, after President Obama's signing of the Plain Writing Act. Similar initiatives have been launched in the UK and Ireland.

The plain language movement is an attempt to demonstrate the benefits of writing clearly and concisely, in a reader-focused style that avoids wordiness, cliché, and jargon. The objective is to write in a style that allows the target audience to readily understand the message, while taking the readers' knowledge of the subject into account. In short, the plain language movement may be called a recipe to use

- a logical organization of your text
- common, everyday words (except for necessary technical terms)
- "we" and other personal pronouns
- the active voice
- short sentences.

People who use documents written in plain language can quickly and easily find what they need, understand what they find, and act on that understanding.

Many scientists believe that they have to write only for colleagues or experts in their own field. An effort to reassess one's own writing style is usually only made after realizing that readers are overwhelmed, overloaded, and too busy to wade through dense writing. Floyd Bloom, MD, former editor of *Science*, has described the attempt to absorb the onslaught of new scientific data as "… like trying to drink from a fire hose. In our bright, new data-packed world, finding the highlights approaches on being an absolute requirement" (Written Communication, March 30, 2002).

Nonetheless, experience proves that scientists are increasingly aware that their journal submissions must adhere to the "Instructions for Authors" of the chosen journal, and most of these clearly encourage plain language. For example, the British Medical Journal (BMJ, see http://www.bmj.com) states, "Please write in a clear, direct, and active style. The BMJ is an international journal, and many readers do not have English as their first language."

Many biomedical communicators would benefit from expanding their reading audience, and they might be surprised how easily this can be achieved. Without any doubt, more medical and scientific breakthroughs will be realized if those additional readers are enlightened or inspired by clear, understandable articles. Moreover, scientists who reach a wider audience might be more successful in persuading policy makers to fund their research. Grant applications written plainly and clearly probably stand a better chance of being funded, assuming, of course, they are worth funding.

> ! Biomedical communicators and scientific writers do not need to "dumb down" scientific writing or omit technical terms to write plainly and clearly. However, they do need to define or explain terms that their audiences may not recognize. They also need to write logically, building from what information the reader knows to what new information the reader will learn in the article.

2.3 The BASO Pyramid of Scientific Writing

As a teacher of scientific writing, I like to use a visual model – a model I have termed the BASO pyramid (an acronym formed from the first letter(s) of **Ba**seline, **S**tyle, and **O**pinion) – to illustrate the various levels of language in science. Let me explain the reasoning behind this.

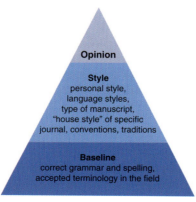

2.3.1 Baseline

Clearly, adherence to the rules of grammar and spelling, as well as the use of the appropriate terminology in the relevant scientific field, must be considered "baseline." In other words, we owe it to the ethics of writing to observe the fundamentals of proper communication, particularly if we communicate in writing. Misspelled words not only confuse – they often annoy the readers to the extent they no longer wish to read the full text. Moreover, poor grammar and erroneous use of technical or scientific terms will jeopardize the credibility of our results. By extrapolation, it is our credibility as scientists that is at stake.

2.3.2 Style

The second level of the BASO pyramid is "style." On this level of writing, we have a certain degree of flexibility and individual freedom, as long as the style we use is compatible with the appropriate guidelines or conventions.

The chosen language inevitably influences the style of scientific writing we use. For example, there are certain differences between American and British usage of English (see also Sect. 3.2). In addition, the type of report or communication we work on will dictate the required style to a certain extent. If we draft a manuscript for publication, the style of writing must be in line with the "house style" of the target journal (see also Sect. 5.5).

Most journals provide some information for authors with respect to the style and structuring of the manuscript intended for submission. Some journals are more specific than others about the style they wish authors to use. Many current journals refer to the *Uniform Requirements for Manuscripts Submitted to Biomedical Journals*: *Writing and Editing for Biomedical Publication* (http://www.icmje.org). This guideline was initially drawn up by a small group of editors of general medical journals in 1978. Because the editors had met informally in Vancouver, British Columbia, they became known as the Vancouver Group (see also Sect. 7.2). Journals that agree to use the *Uniform Requirements* (over 500 do so) are asked to cite the current version of the guidelines in their instructions for authors.

Finally, company-internal conventions or traditions may sometimes influence the style of scientific writing (see also Sect. 5.6). Nowadays, many international pharmaceutical companies use templates for research reports and other documents to ensure homogenous styles and formats across departments and groups. Such style conventions may not necessarily be in full compliance with the generally accepted principles of good scientific writing, but the company staff would be expected to adhere to them. For example, one company may opt for a noncapitalized heading style in their documents, while another may encourage the use of capitals in all titles within a report (see also Sect. 3.6.3).

2.3.3 Opinion

The tip of the BASO pyramid I have termed "opinion." It is important to realize that there is, in fact, room for personal opinion even in the context of scientific writing. This implies that certain issues are not simply "correct" or "incorrect." A particular word may be preferred over another, but the less preferable term may not be wrong as such. Let us consider the following sentences:

> - In this study, we took blood samples immediately *before* starting the infusion.
> In this study, we took blood samples immediately *prior to* starting the infusion.

Is "before" or "prior to" correct here? Clearly, both terms are correct, and the choice solely depends on your personal preference. American writers may go for "prior to," while European writers may favor the more commonly used "before." The same applies to terms such as "following" and "after." Again, the two terms can be used interchangeably in principle, but my advice is to use "after" instead of "following" for two reasons, i.e., the term "after" is shorter, and "following" is used far too often in scientific writing because of its various meanings.

In conclusion, we should always keep in mind that excessive arguing about the "rights" and "wrongs" of scientific writing is a poor investment of precious time, especially if the issue is simply a question of personal opinion.

2.4 Common Myths and Misconceptions

2.4.1 What Are Myths and Misconceptions?

Can we speak of "common misconceptions" in a field as broad and diverse as scientific writing? Is it really possible to find general myths among scientific communicators worldwide who are, inevitably, of many different language origins? The answer is yes; we do find a trend towards general misconceptions that seem to have been passed on by way of tradition in many an institution all over the world. In addition to the "generic" misconceptions we encounter in the scientific and medical literature, there are the more specific difficulties arising from confusion between different languages, such as German and English, for example.

Here are the most frequent shortcomings of scientific texts resulting from myths and misconceptions:

- long and complicated sentences instead of short, clear sentences (Germanic strings of words)
- mixing creative and scientific writing
- scientific "story" not readily apparent
- poor structuring of text by avoiding the use of subheadings
- mixing actual results and their discussion
- inconsistent use of technical terms and units
- misusing or wasting specific and generic terms

- reluctance to use first-person pronouns leading to overuse of passive voice
- tendency to turn sharp and powerful verbs into weighty nouns.

Let us consider some of these aspects in more detail:

2.4.2 Long and Complicated Sentences

Unnecessary words and superfluous decoration of scientific statements obscure the key messages. Thus, readers will find it difficult to grasp the purpose and results of the study. Although current guidelines consistently stress the importance of brevity in scientific reporting, the myth that quantity comes before quality has not yet been eradicated.

The temptation to use ample decoration also comes from the mixing of creative and scientific writing (see also Sect. 5.4). Many scientific authors hold a firm belief that sentences crowded with information add value to their scientific message, and yet they achieve the opposite. Although this problem is evident across the entire scientific literature, it is clearly more pronounced among authors with a language background other than English, such as German or French, for example. I have termed this phenomenon the "Thomas Mann urge," i.e., the urge to be more colorful and flowery than is useful in scientific reporting.

Consider this sentence:

> ● The potentially superior antiplaque and better surface-active properties of amine fluoride and stannous fluoride containing mouth rinses were carefully investigated in a well-designed double-blind, crossover study in 10 healthy volunteers.

Even the learned reader needs considerable time to digest the information contained in this sentence. Why not simply say:

> ● We investigated the antiplaque and surface-active properties of mouth rinses containing amine fluoride and stannous fluoride in a double-blind, crossover study in 10 healthy volunteers.

> ! Quantity can never replace quality of our scientific message, nor can it mask any vagueness we may have because of an incomplete understanding of the concepts.

2.4.3 Misusing or Wasting Specific and Generic Terms

Misuse or waste of specific and generic terms gets in the way of effective communication. Consider this sentence:

2.4 Common Myths and Misconceptions

> • The response of a variety of new antifungal agents is described in the section below.

The sentence implies that it is the "variety" that shows a response, while, in fact, we clearly mean the "antifungal agents." Such collective nouns are best deleted or replaced by an adjective, such as "many" (see also Sect. 11.4).

2.4.4 Reluctance to Use First-Person Pronouns Leading to Overuse of Passive Voice

Reluctance to use first-person pronouns and the resulting overuse of passive voice cause much debate among scientific communicators. Because the issue is of considerable importance, I have dedicated a full section to it (see Sect. 5.2). Here, I just want to stress the need to reconsider the traditional style of passive reporting and to accept the fact that nowadays the active voice is clearly preferred. Active statements are invariably shorter and help avoid unnecessary guessing as to who is responsible for the work reported.

2.4.5 Tendency to Turn Sharp and Powerful Verbs into Weighty Nouns

Why do we so often use bulky nouns when a sleek and elegant verb would do a much better job? Words commonly used as the noun rather than the verb include examination, analysis, investigation, study, and performance, among many others. Why would anyone prefer this?

> • The investigation of the cytochrome P450-dependent drug metabolism was carried out using a microsomal preparation.

Surely, the sentence below is more graceful:

> • We investigated the cytochrome P450-dependent drug metabolism in a microsomal preparation.

Not only do we get rid of a greatly overused (and sometimes abused) noun (investigation); we also make the sentence active by using the personal pronoun "we."

Words and Units: Orthography and Punctuation 3

> *"It's the punctilious attention to detail,*
> *in a time when nobody even bothers*
> *to get the spelling of your name right."*
>
> Holly Brubach

3.1 Correct Spelling

3.1.1 Getting Words Right

The spelling of English is erratic and often illogical. Thus, for a non-native speaker of English, correct spelling is difficult to learn and requires constant reading of English-language material and intensive study of the subject. Words in medical, scientific, and technical texts must be spelled correctly (see also Sect. 2.3). Erroneous spelling is a mark of illiteracy or at least carelessness. Even if we accept that good spelling may be a talent not every good scientist can call his or her own, there is no justification for spelling deficiencies.

Spelling is more than just getting words right. We do not only owe it to the readers to furnish them with proper spelling; we also owe it to ourselves as writers. Although "sloppy" writing in modern everyday communication (e.g., e-mails, SMS, or advertisements) has gained broad acceptance in recent years, few scientific professionals would approve of improper spelling in scientific publications. Even though many spelling errors are typing errors that have escaped the attention of the writer and/or editor, misspelled words distract and annoy the reader. More importantly, poor spelling may lead the reader to conclude that our reported results were obtained with equal carelessness. Needless to say, this detracts from the credibility of our findings.

> ! Misspelled words in sciences distract and annoy the reader. The credibility of your work hinges on the proper use of the language.

3.1.2 Using Spell Checkers

Can the spell checker on your computer help? Modern tools have made it possible to screen texts for spelling mistakes and language inconsistencies, but there are clear limitations. Many words used erroneously in a specific context may escape the spell checker because the faulty word may not be misspelled as such (e.g., "on" in place of "one," "how" in place of "who," "loose" in place of "lose," "it's" in place of "its"). The list of such examples is endless and goes beyond the scope of this book. Nonetheless, my advice is to always use the electronic spell checker before releasing a document, however small, but to apply it *in addition* to manual proofreading and never *instead* of it.

> ! Every document that leaves the writer's desk must have undergone careful screening for spelling errors, both by the author/editor and the spell checker.

3.2 Consistent Spelling: American English Versus British English

"Correctness" may sometimes depend on the type of English chosen. Is it "color" or "colour"? Is it "labelled" or "labeled"? Is "hemoglobin" or "haemoglobin" correct? The answer depends on whether you use American or British spelling.

Despite the widespread transfer of expressions between Britain and the USA, there are still some differences in spelling. Identifying and applying the appropriate spelling becomes less troublesome if we consider the word groups typically affected by this difference (see Sect. 11.2). The list shows examples only and is therefore by no means exhaustive.

Although there is a general trend towards American usage, you are free to choose between American and British English in most situations, unless the recipient of your document has specific requirements. Most journals accept British and American English in manuscripts intended for publication, but the language chosen should be the same within a paper. For example, the British Medical Journal (BMJ) stipulates in its house-style guidance that either American or British English is accepted, "depending on the provenance and main target audience of the article" (see www.bmj.com).

Without any doubt, a mixture of British and American English is tiresome and annoying to the reader. Therefore, scientific writers must be aware of these differences and should consult a good dictionary if in doubt.

> ! A mixture of American and British spelling within any one document is both confusing and annoying to the reader.

If you are unsure of the appropriate language for your manuscript, consider the simple rules below:

> ! If you have the choice, use either American or British spelling, but do so consistently. Keep your target audience in mind (European versus international).
>
> If language requirements are defined (e.g., company-internal conventions, journal house style, publishers' requirements), use the given spelling rules consistently.

> Exercise 1

3.3 Punctuation

3.3.1 Proper Use of Punctuation Marks

Contrary to widespread opinion, punctuation rules are important in scientific, medical, and technical reporting. Because punctuation marks are devised to eliminate ambiguities, they should be applied prudently and consistently. Mistakes in punctuation and haphazard use of punctuation marks undercut the authority of the text and therefore compromise the credibility of your work.

Generally speaking, shorter sentences require less punctuation than do longer ones. Since the reader more readily understands shorter sentences (see also Sect. 2.2), it is good advice to limit the length of sentences. This reduces the number of commas and other punctuation marks at the same time.

The most commonly used punctuation marks in scientific texts are the comma and period (called a "full stop" in British English). After a period, there is a single space, contrary to a commonly held view among less experienced writers that two spaces are needed. This notion comes from the days of the manual typewriter where two spaces were, in fact, used after a period.

Other punctuation marks frequently used include the colon, semicolon, hyphen, apostrophe, slash (also called virgule), and brackets and parentheses. Writers must be sure to apply them correctly. Section 11.3 lists the punctuation marks used in scientific texts and shows examples of using them correctly.

The sections below address some punctuation marks that frequently cause problems in scientific texts.

3.3.2 Hyphens and Word Division

The hyphen connects compound words, prefixes, and suffixes. Although hyphens help to prevent ambiguity and clarify meaning, they should be used sparingly and consistently. However, certain compound words always contain hyphens. Such hyphens are called "orthographic." Examples are brother-in-law, free-for-call, or up-to-date.

Hyphens are no longer necessary for prefixes such as intra, inter, pre, post, non, re, and sub, unless the prefix ends with a vowel and the main word starts with a vowel, e.g., anti-inflammatory, pre-examination, re-analyzed (see also Sect. 11.3). The rules below describe some other situations where you should *not* use a hyphen:

> ! Do not hyphenate Latin expressions or non–English-language phrases used in an adjectival sense, e.g., in vivo experiments, a priori argument.
>
> In the text, do not use hyphens to express a range (e.g., 10% to 20% of the substance), except if the range expresses fiscal years or life spans (e.g., the 2003–2005 data set) or if the range is given in parentheses (e.g., mean age was 22 years; [range, 11–32 years]).
>
> Do not hyphenate modifiers in which the second element is a number or letter, e.g., type 2 diabetes, grade A material.

The question about stand-alone prefixes comes up regularly, e.g., when a contrasting nonhyphenated prefix follows. Examples are terms such as pre- and postinfusion heart rate or intra- and intersubject variation. Although there is growing acceptance of such stand-alone prefixes, it is still good advice to spell out the full term. Thus, I prefer pre-infusion and post-infusion heart rate (here, the hyphens are used because two vowels meet in "pre-infusion" and the same format is applied to "post-infusion" for consistency) or intrasubject and intersubject variation.

Hyphens are also used to break a word at the end of a line. However, words that are divided at the right-hand margin are an interruption to the reader, and incorrectly divided words slow the reader down even more. Thus, word division should be limited to obvious word breaks, e.g., in words with prefixes or suffixes and in compound words. Both parts of a divided word should be pronounceable.

If you choose to divide a term, use the "optional hyphen" on your computer, usually [ctrl+hyphen], rather than the standard hyphen or *en* dash (see Sect. 3.3.3). The optional hyphen will allow word breaks only at the end of a line. If the hyphenated term is no longer at the end of a line because information has been added or deleted after hyphenating the term), the hyphen will not appear in print.

> ! Divide words only if necessary, and divide them correctly.

3.3.3 Punctuation Marks Indicating Emotion

A few punctuation marks indicate emotion, suspense, anticipation, or surprise. Because such sensations have no place in science, these punctuation marks should not be used in scientific writing. "Emotional" punctuation marks include the exclamation point, question mark, and dash.

I cannot think of a single situation where an exclamation point would be appropriate in scientific texts. Very occasionally, you may need the question mark, for example, if someone is being quoted.

> ● At each visit, the investigator asked the patient, "Have you experienced any adverse events since the last visit?"

In general, dashes should be used sparingly in scientific texts, but we do have the occasional use for the *en* dash, for example, to indicate relational distinction in a hyphenated term (see Table 3.1). Unfortunately, the *en* dash is often confused with the hyphen, and many unaware writers use them interchangeably. While hyphens are used to connect or split words (see also Sect. 3.3.2), the *en* dash is only used in special cases. Dashes, if used to add supplementary information, are best replaced by a pair of commas or, alternatively, by parentheses (see Sect. 3.3.4).

Table 3.1 shows the four types of dashes that differ in length. The *en* dash is longer than a hyphen but is half the length of the *em* dash.

Table 3.1 The Four Types of Dashes

NAME OF DASH	SYMBOL	APPROPRIATE USE
en dash	–	*The* en *dash shows relational distinction in a hyphenated or compound modifier if one element consists of two words or a hyphenated word, or when the word being modified is a compound. Multiple sclerosis–like symptoms, Krebs-Henseleit–buffered solution, post–World War II, non–English-language journals.*
em dash	—	*Not used in scientific writing because it indicates a sudden interruption or break in thought (see also* Sect. 3.3.3).
2-em dash	——	*Not used in scientific writing.*
3-em dash	———	*Not used in scientific writing.*

3.3.4 Parentheses and Brackets

Parentheses (round brackets) and brackets [square brackets] are internal punctuation marks used to set off additional information, explanation, or direction. In mathematical or chemical expressions, parentheses alert the reader to special functions occurring within. If the parenthetical material is closely related to the main part of the sentence, use commas instead of parentheses.

Parenthetical information within a parenthetical expression goes into brackets.

- (We studied the neurophysiological changes of the aging brain using functional magnetic resonance imaging [fMRI] or positron emission tomography [PET] techniques.)

In mathematical formulas, the trend is to use only parentheses and brackets. The braces used formerly are slowly being phased out, but some authors and journals still retain them. In mathematical equations, parentheses are generally used for the innermost units. If in doubt, consult the current edition of the *AMA Manual of Style*, *The USP Dictionary of USAN and International Drug Names* for drug formularies, or *The Merck Index* for chemical compounds to verify the use of parentheses and brackets.

- $PVt^2 = [PVb^2 + (PVa^2/TR)]/PQ$

Brackets are used also to indicate editorial interpolation within a quotation and to enclose corrections, explanations, or comments in quoted material. Moreover, many scientific journals use brackets to indicate literature references.

- The editor stated that "most publications [authors not named] were of a high standard."

  Many authors have described a link between metabolic syndrome and the subsequent development of diabetes [1, 3, 10].

To avoid adjacent parentheses or brackets, change the second set to parentheses, or vice versa.

- The weakest effect occurred at the lowest dose (10 mg/kg) [Table 3].

3.3.5 Periods in Titles and Academic Degrees

Should there be a period after Mr, Ms, Mrs, Dr, and Prof? And should periods be used in MD, PhD, BSc, MA, and BA? The answer depends on whom you ask.

Omission of a period in Mr, Ms, Mrs, or Dr is justified because these short forms are suspensions (see Sect. 3.4.6). Suspensions are shortened word forms that consist of the first and last letters of the full word, thus rendering the term "suspended" rather than simply abbreviated. In contrast, "Prof." is not a suspension and should therefore be handled as a "true" abbreviation (see Sect. 3.4.2).

While the traditional Anglo-Saxon approach tends to adhere to the rule for suspensions (i.e., omitting the periods), international use of English has led to a more widespread acceptance of periods in social titles such as Mr. and Dr. In principle, you can decide on either style, as long as consistency is being maintained.

Similarly, you can apply or omit periods in academic titles. As scientific English evolves, periods tend to become less popular in shortened word forms (except in true abbreviations, e.g., temp.). There is no definitive rule other than the need to be consistent. Thus, if you opt for PhD, also use BSc, MA, and MD.

Many writers are uncertain about the correct academic degrees, especially with those obtained in non–English-speaking countries. Because academic training systems tend to vary across the borders, it is often difficult to find the exact English translation. Occasionally, it is good advice to retain the degree description in its original language, even if it appears in an English text. In most cases, however, there is an international term that correctly describes the degree in question (see Sect. 11.5).

3.3.6 Apostrophes in Contractions

Contractions are shortened word combinations in which one or several letters are omitted. Examples of contractions are it's, shouldn't, can't, and don't. Contractions are well accepted in informal writing, but they must never be used in formal professional writing. Here, you should always use the noncontracted forms (it is, should not, cannot, and do not).

> ! Never use contractions in medical, scientific, technical, or other professional texts.

3.3.7 Nonbreaking Spaces and Hyphens

In the past, no one cared much if word combinations, such as numbers accompanied by a unit of measurement or hyphenated expressions representing a single word, were separated at the end of a line. Nowadays, scientific writers do not only have to understand what they are writing about; they also have to apply modern typographic conventions. Spaces between terms that should stay together (e.g., 10 mL, 5 h, pH 7) should always be protected by a so-called nonbreaking space. Similarly, hyphenated terms (e.g., 2-way system, 10-fold dilution) that should not be separated are permanently secured by the use of the nonbreaking hyphen.

Both the nonbreaking space and hyphen are inserted via the insert menu on the toolbar of your word processor (insert → symbol → special characters → nonbreaking space or nonbreaking hyphen). Alternatively, you can use the appropriate shortcut keys, usually [ctrl + shift + space] for nonbreaking space and [ctrl + shift + hyphen] for nonbreaking hyphen.

> ! Use nonbreaking spaces and hyphens to avoid inappropriate separation of terms.

> Exercise 2

3.4 Shortened Word Forms in Scientific Writing

3.4.1 Types of Abbreviations

We often use the term "abbreviation" for any shortened word in scientific texts. More correctly, we distinguish between the following shortened forms of words or phrases (Table 3.2):

Table 3.2 Types of Shortened Word Forms

SHORTENED FORMS	EXAMPLES
True abbreviations	*Temp., Prof., approx.*
Units of measurement	*mL, h, s, m, km*
Acronyms	*AIDS, ELISA, NATO, ANOVA*
Initialisms	*HPLC, WHO, ATP, DNA*
Contractions	*Isn't, shouldn't, doesn't, it's* (*see also* Sect. 3.3.6)
Suspensions	*Mr, Ms, Dr, cont'd,* (*see also* Sect. 3.3.5)

Shortened or contracted forms of words or phrases replace the full term. Clearly, the use of such short forms helps to save time, space, and printing cost. Nonetheless, many professional journals discourage the use of shortened word forms or at least limit their number, unless these are well-recognized clinical, technical, or general terms or accepted units of measurement. In any case, obscure abbreviations that are not used internationally should be avoided because they confuse, rather than enlighten, the reader. Similarly, terms that share the same abbreviation (e.g., AHA for American Heart Association and American Hospital Association, or CV for coefficient of variation, cardiovascular, and curriculum vitae) should not be shortened (see also Sect. 3.4.4).

If you are uncertain whether a term is commonly used or not, consult a reliable list of abbreviations (e.g., *AMA Manual of Style* or *CBE Manual for Authors, Editors, and Publishers*).

The following rules apply to all abbreviations used in scientific writing, except units of measurement:

! Define abbreviations the first time they appear. Subsequently, use the abbreviation rather than the full term.

Avoid abbreviations in titles and abstracts, as well as at the beginning of a sentence (unless the full term is cumbersome or excessively lengthy).

Use a glossary of abbreviations (unless this is not encouraged by the journal to which you wish to submit your paper).

3.4.2 True Abbreviations

True abbreviations are those that simply shorten a term (e.g., approx.; see also Sect. 3.3.5). Such short forms are given in lowercase letters unless the full term is a proper name or the abbreviation is the first word in a sentence. Use these short forms sparingly and avoid shortened terms that cause confusion. In tables, figures, or parentheses, abbreviations can be used to save space. However, these must be defined in full, either in a footnote or the legend.

3.4.2.1 Latin Abbreviations

Generally speaking, English terms and abbreviations are preferred to Latin expressions or other foreign words. However, some Latin abbreviations are commonly used in science, preferably confined to parenthetical references. The use of these abbreviations makes sense because they are shorter than their English equivalents.

Commonly used Latin abbreviations include cf. (*confer*, compare), etc. (*et cetera*, and so forth), e.g. (*exempli gratia*, for example), et al. (*et alii*, and others; note that there is a period after al. but not after et), and i.e. (*id est*, that is).

> ● In certain conditions (e.g., endocarditis, foreign-body infections) or infections in immunocompromised patients, bactericidal activity (i.e., the killing of bacteria) is indispensable for clinical cure.

For e.g. and i.e., current conventions generally still recommend the use of periods as shown above, but the trend is towards omitting the periods. Similarly, italics in Latin and other foreign terms are increasingly being avoided. As is true for every situation, the overriding rule is to be consistent and to consult the appropriate house-style recommendations or editorial requirements before finalizing your manuscript.

3.4.3 Units of Measurement

Units of measurement are abbreviated when used with numerical values but are not abbreviated if used without numerical values.

> ● We added NaCl (4 mg). Concentrations are expressed as milligrams of sodium chloride per liter of water.

Use Arabic numerals in combination with units, such as length, weight, percentages, and degrees of temperature. The plural form of units of measurement is the same as the singular form (e.g., 1 mL, 10 mL; 1 h, 10 h). Remember to leave a space between the number and unit, except for the percentage mark that follows the number without a space.

> ● The patients received a daily dose of either 1 mg or 10 mg for 14 days.
>
> The mortality rate in the 6-month toxicity study in rats was 1.2%.

The units and symbols of the International System of Units ("Système International d'Unités", SI) and certain derived SI units have become part of the language of science. This modern metric system should be mastered by all scientific professionals and students. Units of measurement often cause confusion in scientific texts, especially if they are used inconsistently. The problem arises because the SI system does not define all units used commonly in science. The system, based on eight fundamental units of measurement (Lippert and Lehmann 1978), was designed to harmonize the international use of units and to combat confusion and inconsistencies in the traditional metric system. Table 3.3 shows the fundamental SI units of measurement.

Table 3.3 Fundamental SI Units of Measurement

PROPERTY	BASE UNIT	SI SYMBOL
Length	meter	m
Mass	kilogram	kg
Time	second	s
Concentration	molar	M
Amount	mole	mol
Thermodynamic temperature	kelvin	K
Electric current	ampere	A
Luminous intensity	candela	cd

Other units, such as liter or hour, are derived from these base units. Although no definitive symbol exists for these derived units, a simple "h" for hour and an "L" for liter are nowadays standard. The "L" for liter may or may not be capitalized, although the capital L is gaining broader acceptance. Make sure to use the same symbol for units containing "L," e.g., µL, mL, or dL. Table 3.4 shows the standard SI prefixes to express multiples.

Table 3.4 Standard SI Prefixes

FACTOR	SI PREFIX	SYMBOL
10^{18}	exa-	E
10^{15}	peta-	P
10^{12}	tera-	T
10^{9}	giga-	G
10^{6}	mega-	M
10^{3}	kilo-	k
10^{-3}	milli-	m
10^{-6}	micro-	µ
10^{-9}	nano-	n
10^{-12}	pico-	p
10^{-15}	femto-	f
10^{-18}	atto-	a

> ! Use units of measurement consistently (e.g., ml or mL).
>
> Use the same abbreviations for the singular and plural forms (e.g., 1 mL, 10 mL; 1 h, 3 h; 1 cm, 50 cm).

3.4.4 Acronyms and Initialisms

An acronym is a word formed from the initial letters or groups of letters of words in a set phrase or series of words. Acronyms are pronounced as words. Similarly, initialisms are built from the first letters of a group of words, but here, each letter is pronounced separately.

In scientific writing, acronyms and initialisms are handled in the same way. Generally speaking, they should be used sparingly (usually only for terms mentioned at least five times in any text). However, this may depend on the guidelines or house style of the relevant organization or journal for which the manuscript is being written. In any case, obscure acronyms or initialisms that are not internationally used should be avoided (see also Sect. 3.4.1).

Here are the rules governing the use of acronyms and initialisms:

> ! Use capitals and no periods (full stops) for acronyms and initialisms. Exceptions are terms that have become commonly accepted as nouns (e.g., laser, scuba).
>
> Do not capitalize the words from which an acronym or initialism is derived (e.g., prostate-specific antigen [PSA]).
>
> Use no apostrophe in plural forms (e.g., ECGs, RBCs).

In texts and reports other than manuscripts intended for publication in a scientific journal, you should provide a glossary of abbreviations. A glossary allows the reader to quickly access the full term if there is uncertainty. However, a glossary never replaces the introduction of the abbreviated term in the text; it is provided in addition to the individual definitions rather than instead.

3.4.5 Contractions

Contractions are shortened word combinations in which one or more letters are omitted (e.g., it's, shouldn't, don't). As pointed out in Sect. 3.3.6, contractions are well accepted in speech or informal writing, but they have no place in formal professional writing. Thus, the correct forms in formal writing are "it is, should not, do not," etc.

3.4.6 Suspensions

Suspensions are shortened word forms that consist of the first and last letters of the full word. Examples are titles of persons (e.g., Mr, Ms, Mrs, and Dr) commonly used in combination with the full name, for example, Dr Albert Schweitzer (see also Sect. 3.3.5). Earlier, the distinction between true abbreviations (e.g., Prof., requiring a period) and suspensions (e.g., Mr, not requiring a period) reflected British usage of the English language, but nowadays, the general move towards using periods in "Mr." and "Dr." is becoming increasingly widespread.

> ! Suspensions (e.g., Mr, Dr) do not have to be followed by a period. True abbreviations (e.g., Prof.), however, always end with a period.

3.5 Numbers

3.5.1 Expressing Numbers in Scientific Texts

Numbers play an important role in scientific communication. Most scientific texts contain numbers, and in many types of texts, such as clinical or statistical reports, numbers may even predominate over simple words. Therefore, it is of utmost importance to express numbers in a consistent and logical manner.

> ! Getting your numbers right first time saves much time and effort in subsequent editing rounds.

Unfortunately, rules for writing numbers tend to vary between sources, which complicates the issue to some extent. Rules depend not only on the type of manuscript in preparation but also on the body making the rule. Moreover, conventions in number expression are changing as time goes on. A conservative rule that many editors and writing experts still recommend is this:

> ! Spell out one-digit numbers (one to nine), and use numerals for all larger numbers.

Table 3.5 shows some exceptions.

3.5 Numbers

Table 3.5 Spelling Numbers Correctly

WHERE	HOW
At the beginning of a sentence	Spell out numbers at the beginning of a sentence. With very large numbers, rearrange the sentence in such a way that the number is no longer at the beginning.
With units of measurement	Always use numerals if a unit of measurement follows (e.g., 3 mL, 9 h, 5 min).
In a series	In a series, use numerals if any number in the series is 10 or larger (e.g., In total, 2 monkeys, 5 rabbits, and 12 rats were used).
If two numbers appear back to back	If two numbers appear back to back, write one out (e.g., ten 20-mg doses).

An increasing number of international journals now use numerals (Arabic numbers) throughout, even for very small numbers. This trend is expected to continue in an effort to shorten texts and reduce printing costs. Therefore, it is important to consult the guidelines of the editor/organizer in question before starting to write.

Terms such as "billion," "trillion," and "quadrillion" should be avoided because they mean different numbers in Europe and the USA.

In narrative sections of a manuscript, try to avoid powers of 10 as they can be difficult to interpret. However, there are situations where powers make sense because this is shorter, e.g., in tables, figures, or parenthetical information, as shown in the example below:

● Sales were substantially higher in 2013 than last year (i.e., 1.2×10^9 units versus 0.8×10^9 units sold in 2012).

! Whatever style of expressing numbers you adopt, remember to be consistent. Heterogeneous styles in any single document are both distracting and annoying to the reader.

3.5.2 Formats of Numbers

Decimal points and thousands create much confusion in scientific writing because of the divergent styles used in different languages. A particular problem is the decimal point that is used differently in English and German. In English, a comma denotes thousands, while in German the comma stands for the decimal point.

Much effort has gone into finding an international style for thousands and fractions of numbers. Although the attempt to globalize these styles is honorable, it has not (yet) led to universally accepted conventions. My advice is to use the traditional British/American approach unless the editor/publisher or other organization has made specific provisions. Table 3.6 shows the European, traditional Anglo-Saxon, and suggested international styles.

Table 3.6 Thousands and Decimal Points

EUROPEAN	TRADITIONAL BRITISH AND AMERICAN	RECOMMENDED FOR INTERNATIONAL SCIENTIFIC REPORTING
1'000	1,000 or 1000	1000
2'568	2,568 or 2568	2568
47 938, 275	47,938.275	47 938.275
0,525	0.525	0.525 (*always give "0" before the decimal point*)
$P=0{,}05$	$P=0.05$	$P=0.05$

3.5.3 Ranges of Numbers

Table 3.7 shows how to express ranges in texts, tables, parentheses, and references.

Table 3.7 Expressing Ranges

RANGES	HOW TO EXPRESS	COMMENTS
In texts	*Samples 38 to 45 were scanned at wavelengths from 240 nm to 350 nm.* *1938 to 1968*	Use the words "to" or "through" (American) rather than a dash in texts (*see also Sect. 3.3.2*).
In tables, parentheses, and references	*samples 38–45* *see 3.2–3.7* *pp. 224–248* *1938–1968*	Use an *en* dash or hyphen. In literature references, duplicate numbers are sometimes omitted (e.g., *pp. 224–48*).

3.5.4 Percentages

The terms "percent," "percentage," and "percentile" cause considerable confusion in scientific texts because they are often used erroneously. "Percent," sometimes written "per cent," means in, to, or for every hundred. A number should always precede "percent." The term "percentage," however, implies a number or amount expressed in percent. Percentile is a statistical term for the value in a distribution of frequencies divided into 100 equal groups. Table 3.8 shows the correct use of these terms.

Table 3.8 Expressing Percentages Correctly

PERCENT, PERCENTAGES, AND PERCENTILES	EXAMPLE	COMMENTS
Percent ranges	*The success rate was 15% to 47%.*	There is no space between the number and the percent symbol. Repeat the percent symbol for each number in a series or range, even for zero.
Percent in a series	*The purities in the three batches amounted to 88%, 69%, and 99%.*	Repeat the symbol for each number.
Percent at the beginning of a sentence	*Fifty-seven percent of patients were free of symptoms.*	Spell out both the number and the word "percent." Alternatively, rearrange the sentence. Use the plural "were" because *57% implies 57 samples of 100 samples.*

(continued)

3.6 Capitalization

Table 3.8 (continued)

PERCENT, PERCENTAGES, AND PERCENTILES	EXAMPLE	COMMENTS
Percentages	The percentage of failures was higher in the current study.	"Percentage" implies the number of failures expressed in percent.
Percentiles	The boy's growth rate was at the 99th percentile.	Do not confuse "percentile" with "percentage."

In clinical reporting, it may be more meaningful to give the actual number of subjects or patients if the population includes fewer than 50 subjects. Sometimes, the actual number is followed by the percentage in parentheses. Decimals in percentages should only be used if the 100% value is higher than 1000.

> ● Serious adverse events occurred in 5 (10%) patients. Of the 1278 patients participating, 37 (2.9%) did not respond to treatment.

> Exercise 3

3.6 Capitalization

3.6.1 Use of Capitals in Scientific English

The English language uses capitals sparingly. In scientific writing, there has been a trend over time to use fewer capitals rather than more. However, usage varies, depending on the journal's house style, company-internal conventions, and predefined document standards. Before submitting a manuscript, consult the appropriate style requirements.

Generally, the only rule we have to know is this:

> ! Capitalized words in science are either proper nouns, key words in titles, or first words of sentences.

3.6.2 Capitals in Proper Nouns (Names)

Proper nouns designate a specific person, place, thing, or idea. Thus, proper nouns are names. All proper nouns are capitalized, as is any word derived from them (e.g., Alzheimer's disease, Dalton's law). The rule seems easy enough – why then is it that authors often find it hard to use proper capitalization?

Many common nouns we use in science could easily be mistaken for proper nouns and writers may be tempted to capitalize them. These include chemicals, generic drug names, microorganisms, diseases, physiological processes, or common names derived from the scientific names of plants and animals. Table 3.9 shows examples of proper and common nouns.

Table 3.9 Examples of Proper and Common Nouns

PROPER NOUNS	COMMON NOUNS
Xerox machine	*photocopier*
Dacron	*synthetic polyester*
Novocain	*procaine*
Aspirin®	*aspirin*
IMx Rubella test	*rubella*
Celsius (*a scientist's name*)	*centigrade*
Asperger autism	*autistic disorder*
Parkinson's disease	*parkinsonism*
Wistar rats	*transgenic rats*
Alsatian dogs	*beagle dogs*
Staphylococcus aureus	*staphylococci*
Neisseria gonorrheae	*gonococcus*
Plasmodium falciparum	*malarial parasite*

3.6.3 Capitals in Titles

In titles, you may capitalize the so-called important words to add emphasis. If you opt for capitalization in titles, capitalize nouns, adjectives, pronouns, verbs, numerals, and adverbs. Do not capitalize articles, conjunctions, and prepositions. Sometimes, prepositions or conjunctions containing five or more letters (e.g., above, underneath) are also capitalized. If this is the style you use, make sure to be consistent.

> ● Pharmacokinetic Parameters of the Parent Compound and the Three Metabolites in Plasma of Rats, Rabbits, and Monkeys

3.6.3.1 Capitalizing Hyphenated Compound Words in Titles

In titles, subtitles, and headings of tables or figures, capitalize both terms in compound words unless one part of the word combination is a prefix or suffix, or if both words together constitute a single word (if in doubt about hyphenating such terms, consult the current edition of *Merriam-Webster's Collegiate Dictionary* or *Dorland's Medical Dictionary*). Consider the following examples:

> ● Placebo-Controlled Study, Event-Related Potential, Aspirin-Treated Subjects, Low-Level Radioactivity (both terms capitalized)
>
> Anti-infective Drugs, Intra-arterial Embolism, Intra-assay Precision (second part of compound not capitalized because of prefix)
>
> Follow-up Studies, Short-term Analysis, X-ray Examination (second part of compound not capitalized because of single-word meaning)

3.6.4 Capitals in Designations

In designations, capitalize terms such as table, figure, and appendix if they are accompanied by a number.

> ● As indicated, Table 5 summarizes the demographic data. For individual data consult Appendix 2.

However, some words are not capitalized even when used as specific designations, unless they are part of a title (Table 3.10).

Table 3.10 Words Not Capitalized if Used as Designators

NONCAPITALIZED DESIGNATORS			
axis	experiment	method	schedule
case	factor	month	section
chapter	fraction	notes	series
chromosome	grade	page	stage
column	grant	paragraph	step
control	group	part	type
day	lead	patient	volume
edition	level	phase	week

From AMA Manual of Style: A Guide for Authors and Editors. 10th ed. Oxford University Press; 2009.

3.6.5 Capitals in New-Age Words

A frequent question is whether modern words, such as "e-mail," should start with a capital letter. Although the New York Times initially recommended a capital "E" in their Manual of Style and Usage, e-mail (lowercased) has become the favored style all over the world. The argument is that the term has meanwhile become a household expression and would therefore no longer qualify as a proper noun. Even italicizing is no longer necessary, owing to the broad exposure of the term. Again, this is a nice example of linguistic evolution that takes into account common usage of modern words.

> ● He had to change his e-mail address because of the many SPAMs sent to his account.

> > Exercise 4

Forming Sentences: Grammar   4

> *"There's a great power in words,*
> *if you don't hitch too many of them together."*
>
> Josh Billings

4.1 Why Battle with Grammar?

We may know much about the proper structuring of a paper and correct spelling of words, but this does not suffice to produce a compelling manuscript. Ultimately, the power of our text hinges on the competent use of the English language. If your native tongue does not happen to be English, using proper and powerful grammar may be more difficult, but even if you are a native English speaker, you may occasionally struggle with English grammar and its proper use in scientific writing.

Sometimes, students of scientific writing point out that it is hardly worth their while to pay close attention to grammatical detail, knowing that few readers will appreciate their special effort and that most will have a language origin other than English. While there is some truth in this, I would argue that it is precisely for this very reason, i.e., just *because* many readers are non-native English speakers, that we owe it to the scientific community to write in a clear and unambiguous style. Remember that the main purpose of communicating within the sciences is to pass on pertinent information that is read and understood by the intended audience.

As I have pointed out in earlier sections, this book is not about English grammar as such. There are many excellent books on English grammar and usage that you may wish to consult if you have specific questions. When talking about grammar in workshops and lectures, students often point out some basic rules of English grammar they remember from their school days. What about splitting infinitives? Can we end a sentence with a preposition? Do singular subjects always take singular verbs? The good news is that most of these basic rules of grammar are outdated and have little value in scientific English. The most important rule of grammar in scientific communication is to convey meaning to the reader. A clear sentence is a good sentence, even if so-called rules have been broken. Conversely, you may produce a sentence with impeccable grammar that means absolutely nothing to the reader.

Here, our focus is clearly on the use of the English language to convey scientific messages to the learned audience. Because good scientific writing requires proper use of the English language, we will, however, have to look at some aspects of grammar. This section addresses some typical questions of grammar and usage in connection with scientific writing. The section is by no means exhaustive; it merely focuses on the topics I consider most troublesome and whose proper handling will add the greatest power to your scientific messages.

Table 4.1 defines the main grammatical elements we use in scientific reporting. Consulting this table may help when a specific word type or other structure needs to be identified.

Table 4.1 Grammar in Brief

STRUCTURE	DESCRIPTION
Sentence	Grammatical construction containing a subject and an action
Subject	Responsible for the action in a sentence
Noun	Word naming a concrete (e.g., book) or abstract (e.g., love) thing
Pronoun	Word replacing a noun (e.g., he, she, that)
Modifier	Adjective (modifying a noun), adverb (modifying an adjective or a verb), or noun (modifying another noun)
Phrase	Group of words acting as a noun or modifier
Clause	Group of words acting as a noun or modifier, containing a subject and a verb (in contrast to a phrase)
Metaphor/simile	Word or image used to describe something not like itself (e.g., the "head" of a company)

4.2 The Tenses in Scientific Reporting

I usually start my lecture on the tenses in scientific reporting by reassuring my students and workshop participants that "there is no need to get tense about the tense." We just need to know a few rules governing the correct handling of the tenses.

Proper use of tense in scientific documents derives from scientific ethics, i.e., we owe it to the scientific community to declare, by the choice of tense, whether we report established facts or new, previously unpublished data. When a scientific paper has been published in a primary journal (i.e., a journal that publishes only original data), the information communicated becomes "established knowledge." This definition often creates heated discussion among my students as they point out, quite rightly, that so many a published "fact" will prove untrue in subsequent studies. In this respect, "established knowledge" occasionally turns out to be a transient phenomenon. Nonetheless, validly published findings are regarded as "knowledge" as long as the findings have not been challenged or even disproved elsewhere.

4.2 The Tenses in Scientific Reporting

Let me reassure you that you will hardly ever encounter the situation where the distinction between established knowledge and new results presents a problem. When you describe the scientific context of your work, for example the disease your work deals with, you will automatically use the present tense to detail what is known about the incidence, prevalence, cause, and perhaps therapy of the disease in question.

> ● *Established knowledge*: HIV infection **is** highly prevalent in African countries [12].
>
> *Your own new finding*: Inhibition of the enzyme **resulted** in much higher plasma levels of the parent drug.
>
> *When referring to your finding after its publication*: Inhibition of the enzyme **results** in much higher plasma levels of the parent drug [2].

Therefore, the two tenses mainly used in scientific writing are the simple present and the simple past. The so-called perfect tenses (e.g., have been, had been) should be used sparingly. The perfect tenses are appropriate only if we refer to a moment in time before the reporting time point (requiring the past perfect) or if we describe a state of progression or a situation that is still persisting (requiring the present perfect).

> ● Immediately after puncturing, a stopwatch was started and the blood absorbed every 10–15 s using the edge of a piece of filter paper until all visible bleeding **had ceased**. (Past perfect)
>
> Only those mice that **had** previously **been injected** with the study drug were included in the experiment. (Past perfect)
>
> The Department of Physiology **has been located** in Building 221 since 1985. (Present perfect)

Thus, the rule to remember is this:

> ! Report established knowledge in the present tense but new, previously unpublished findings (including your own results) in the past tense.

Difficulties often arise when referring to attributions or data presentations (see Table 4.2). It is correct to say, "Miller [10] *showed* that the cure rate in infected outpatients *is* approx. 15%." In your manuscript or report, it is also correct to say, "Figure 1 *indicates* that younger subjects *had* a higher chance of responding to treatment."

Table 4.2 shows the tense appropriate in a specific context or section of a scientific manuscript.

Table 4.2 Rules for Applying the Appropriate Tense

CONTEXT OR SECTION	APPROPRIATE TENSE
Established knowledge, previous results, etc.	*Present tense*
Methods, materials used, and results	*Past tense*
Description of tables and figures	*Present tense, e.g., Table 5 shows…; Figure 2 illustrates…*
Attribution	*Past tense, e.g., Jones et al. reported that…; Davies found…*

In a typical scientific paper, correct use of these rules will inevitably result in switching of tenses, sometimes within the same section. Many writers wrongly assume that the same tense, e.g., the present tense or past tense, should be applied to the entire manuscript or report. With the distinction between established and new findings in mind, this is clearly not possible, nor would it be correct.

Choosing the correct tense is hardest in the Discussion section. Here, we may emphasize the relationship of our work to previously established knowledge, using attribution to other workers and referring to reported findings. Moreover, we may express a personal opinion, which should be in the present tense (e.g., "We feel that these findings indicate…"; "It is our opinion…"; "We emphasize that…"). Occasionally, there may be a need to announce further actions (e.g., "We plan to investigate this phenomenon in a larger study…"). As a general rule, future work should be mentioned with caution because so many planned (and promised) experiments and studies never actually get off the ground.

Table 4.3 shows the tenses predominantly used in the various sections of a paper or report. Clearly, there may be a switch from the present to the past, and vice versa, even within individual sections of a paper. If we let common sense prevail, we can avoid most errors in the choice of the appropriate tense.

Table 4.3 Tenses Typically Occurring in a Paper or Report

SECTION	PREDOMINANT TENSE
Abstract / Summary	*Past*
Introduction	*Mostly present tense (established facts, previously published data)*
Materials / Methods	*Past*
Results	*Past*
Discussion / Conclusions	*Mixture of past and present, sometimes future tense*

> Exercise 5

4.3 Joining Statements

4.3.1 How Can the Joining of Words or Statements Cause Confusion?

Confused scientific writing often comes about by erroneously joining sentences, clauses, or even single terms. The resulting incoherence is called "nonparallelism." I would argue that nonparallelism is, indeed, responsible for many errors, some of which are serious enough to lead the reader to draw the wrong conclusions. Nonparallel statements often come about because we think faster than we write or because we expect the reader to deduce the correct message from our statements although the text is unclear. Another reason for the many nonparallel sentences in science is carelessness, an attitude grossly incompatible with the enormous precision we exercise when doing scientific work. Please bear in mind that it is unfair to the readers of our paper to let them guess what we were trying to say.

Nonparallel statements may occur on all levels of a sentence, for example when joining nouns, verbs, modifiers, prepositional phrases, or entire sentences. The joining words are called conjunctions, and these may be of the coordinating or subordinating type (Table 4.4). Coordinating conjunctions join terms that are equals, whereas subordinating conjunctions show inequality or a relationship of dependence or limitation. Both types of conjunctions may be involved in nonparallel constructions.

4.3.2 Nonparallel Verbs

Table 4.4 The Two Types of Conjunctions

TYPE	EXAMPLES
Coordinating	*and, or, but, for, nor, so, yet*
Subordinating	*if, as, when, because*

Let us consider some nonparallel statements typically occurring in scientific or medical reporting:

● *Incorrect*: The department was responsible for recruiting, monitoring, and analyzing the data.

This sentence implies that "data" were recruited and monitored, when, in fact, it was the patients who were recruited and the trial that was monitored. The sentence should be reworded to make this clear:

● *Correct*: The department was responsible for recruiting the patients, monitoring the trial, and analyzing the data.

Another source of nonparallel statements is the change of verb number within the sentence:

● *Incorrect*: A small volume of water was added to the mixture and the samples incubated for 24 h.

Here, the second verb should be "were," but this was simply skipped. The second verb can only be omitted if the verb number (i.e., singular or plural) is the same.

- *Correct*: A small volume of water was added to the mixture, and the samples were incubated for 24 h.

Joining transitive and intransitive verbs can also lead us astray:

- *Incorrect*: Her publication on current therapies far surpasses and is clearly superior to previously published reviews.

Here, the transitive verb "surpasses" requires an object and therefore cannot stand alone. The assumed object in this example is "published reviews," but it is incorrect to join the transitive verb (surpass) and the intransitive verb (is) via the conjunction "and." This is one way of correcting the sentence:

- *Correct*: Her publication on current therapies far surpasses any previously published reviews and is clearly superior to the available reports in the literature.

We have restored grammatical parallelism, but the style of the sentence may be questioned because to surpass something and to be superior to it is a tautology (see also Sect. 6.3). I suggest the following:

- *Correct and preferred*: Her publication on current therapies is far superior to any previously published reviews.

4.3.3 Nonparallel Modifiers

Lack of parallelism often occurs when comparing things:

- *Incorrect*: In this study, the new compound was as efficacious but safer than the comparator drug.

Here, "efficacious" is erroneously linked with "than." The term should have read "as efficacious as the comparator drug" to restore grammatical parallelism. We may overcome this lack of parallelism by rewording the sentence:

- *Correct*: In this study, the new compound was as efficacious as the comparator drug and was safer.

4.3.4 Nonparallel Prepositional Phrases

When joining prepositional phrases, the temptation to produce a nonparallel sentence appears to be overwhelming.

> ● *Incorrect*: These templates are for your clinical staff, and for when they plan to design a large clinical study.

This sentence raises questions. Are the templates for all members of your clinical staff or just for those who plan to design a large clinical study? Are the templates of general use, or are they just suitable for the design of large clinical studies? Well, we could speculate on the intended meaning of the sentence for hours and would still not know for sure.

Here is another troublesome statement suffering from a nonparallel structure:

> ● *Incorrect*: We developed this novel laxative for patients with hemorrhoids, anal fissures, and after surgery.

Do we have the correct number of "ands" in this sentence? We can easily see that the first part of this compound sentence "We developed this novel laxative *for patients with hemorrhoids, anal fissures*" is incomplete. In parallel sentences, each clause should be able to stand independently. The sentence can be cured of its nonparallel structure by adding the missing "and" and repeating the object of the sentence (i.e., "patients").

> ● *Correct*: We developed this novel laxative for patients with hemorrhoids and anal fissures, and for patients who have undergone surgery.

> ! For parallelism, the terms linked via a conjunction must have the same grammatical structure.

> \> Exercise 6

4.4 Subject–Verb Agreement

4.4.1 Using the Correct Verb Forms

It is important for writers to pay attention to subject–verb agreement because errors can lead to gross confusion. In principle, the story is a simple one: a singular subject takes a singular verb, and a plural subject takes a plural verb.

This simple rule works in most cases and should therefore be followed wherever appropriate.

- *Correct*: The study **shows** the importance of measuring blood concentrations at the specified intervals.
  Correct: The studies **show** the importance of measuring blood concentrations at the specified intervals.

One of the problems is that we are often unsure of the subject in the sentence, especially if the sentence is long and the verb is far removed from its subject. Sometimes, such sentences can be cured of their lack of subject–verb agreement by rearranging the syntax.

- *Incorrect*: The generation of excessively large sets of data were responsible for the delay in finalizing the study.
  Incorrect: The effects of alcohol on enzyme induction was studied in vitro.

The subject of the first sentence is "generation," a singular noun requiring a singular verb (i.e., was). In the second sentence, the subject is plural (i.e., "effects"); thus, the plural "were" is required. If in doubt, temporarily ignore all phrases between the subject and verb, and the actual sentence becomes readily apparent.

- *Correct*: The generation of…data was responsible for the delay in finalizing the study.
  Correct: The effects…were studied in vitro.

Another frequent problem is the erroneous use of plural terms. Many writers use plural words as singular nouns, not realizing that these terms have, in fact, a matching singular form. Table 4.5 shows some typical examples of plurals erroneously used as singulars.

Table 4.5 Erroneous Use of Plural Nouns

INCORRECT	CORRECT
The main study criteria was the reduction in death rate at the end of the 3-month treatment period.	*The main study criterion was the reduction in death rate at the end of the 3-month treatment period.*
The data was analyzed descriptively.	*The data were analyzed descriptively.*
The causative bacteria was identified.	*The causative bacteria were identified.*
The media used in the incubation experiments was free of glucose.	*The medium used in the incubation experiments was free of glucose.* Or (*if several media were used*): *The media used in the incubation experiments were free of glucose.*
This phenomena warrants further study.	*This phenomenon warrants further study.*

4.4 Subject–Verb Agreement

> ! In general, a singular subject takes a singular verb, and a plural subject takes a plural verb.

4.4.2 Special Nouns

A few nouns are plural in form but singular in meaning (e.g., news). Other nouns have no plural form and therefore always take the singular verb (e.g., information). Moreover, some singular nouns look like plurals because of their "s" at the end (e.g., measles or mumps). Table 4.6 shows examples and correct use of such special nouns.

Table 4.6 Using Special Nouns Correctly

SPECIAL NOUN	CORRECT USE
News	This is news to me.
Information	Information on patient compliance was collected during the study.
Measles	Nowadays, measles is rare in Western countries.
Mumps	Mumps is often accompanied by complications.

4.4.3 Collective Nouns

While most nouns are clearly either singular or plural in both sense and form, there are some exceptions that may cause difficulties. A collective noun indicates a group or collection of persons, organizations, things, or qualities. Table 4.7 shows some typical collective nouns.

Table 4.7 Typical Collective Nouns

TYPE OF COLLECTIVE NOUN	EXAMPLES
Groups of people	audience, public, staff, personnel, crew, class, couple, team, congregation, delegation
Organizations	police, government, army, faculty
Things (e.g., data)	percent, majority
Qualities / disciplines	genetics, pharmacokinetics, statistics, toxicokinetics, genomics, mathematics

The general rule is that such nouns are plural in meaning but singular in form.

> ● The audience was delighted with the performance.
> The personnel plans to go on strike because of the pay cut.

However, if the individual members of a group or constituents of a collection are emphasized, the plural verb is correct. Table 4.8 shows examples of collective nouns that can be either singular or plural in meaning.

Table 4.8 Collective Nouns with Both Singular and Plural Forms

SINGULAR FORM	PLURAL FORM
The couple needs counseling. (Couple is considered a unit; thus, the singular verb is appropriate.)	The couple work at two different hospitals. (Couple is regarded as the two individuals, rather than a unit; thus, the plural verb is appropriate.)
The police is an important institution. (Police is considered an organization; thus, the singular verb is appropriate.)	The police were quick to respond to the alarm. (Police refers to the individual members rather than the organization as a whole; thus, the plural verb is appropriate.)
The faculty has recently been reformed. (Faculty is considered a unit; thus, the singular verb is appropriate.)	The faculty come from many different areas. (Faculty refers to the individual members rather than the group as a whole; thus, the plural verb is appropriate.)
The majority of his time goes into report writing. (Majority is considered an amount; thus, the singular verb is appropriate.)	The majority of results were correct. (Majority refers to the individual results rather than the collection as a whole; thus, the plural verb is appropriate.)
Ten percent of her income goes to the research foundation. (Ten percent is regarded as an amount; thus, the singular verb is appropriate.)	Ten percent of the staff work flexible hours. (Ten percent is regarded as composed of each individual staff member; thus, the plural verb is appropriate.)
Genetics is a popular field of research nowadays. (Genetics is regarded as a discipline; thus, the singular verb is appropriate.)	The genetics of the fruit fly were elucidated in our laboratory. (Genetics refers to the individual findings; thus, the plural verb is appropriate.)

4.4.4 The Rule of Meaning

Some mass nouns, e.g., "total" and "number," are particularly difficult to handle. When the total or number referred to indicates a single quantity, entity, or unit, these terms take the singular verb. If, however, the individual components of the total or number are concerned, you should use the plural verb. Essentially, we place meaning before grammatical correctness in such cases. Table 4.9 shows some typical examples of mass nouns, used with either the singular or plural verb depending on meaning.

Table 4.9 The Rule of Meaning Applied Properly

SINGLE VERB REQUIRED	PLURAL VERB REQUIRED (RULE OF MEANING)
A total of 20 g of calcium sulfate was added. (Single quantity)	A total of 41 patients were enrolled in the study. (Total implies individual patients.)
A total of 200 mL of blood was collected. (Single volume)	A number of data were statistically significant. (Number implies individual data.)

4.4 Subject–Verb Agreement

Many writers feel uncomfortable with the terms "a total of" or "a number of." Often, it is good advice to rewrite such sentences and replace the troublesome collective noun as shown below.

- Calcium sulfate (20 g) was added.
  The total volume of blood collected amounted to 200 mL.
  Overall, 41 patients were enrolled in the study.
  Some data were statistically significant.

If the definite article accompanies "total" or "number," the term always takes a singular verb.

- The number of participating centers was 12.
  The total of returned questionnaires was 130.

! For terms that can be either singular or plural, use the singular verb if the term refers to a unit, amount, discipline, or organization. Use the plural verb if the term indicates individual members or components rather than the collection as a whole.

4.4.5 Verb Matching with "None" and the "Neither–Nor" Linkage

"None" can mean "not any" or "not one." If "none" specifically means "not any," a plural verb is preferable:

- None of the experiments were able to produce the intended results.

If "none" clearly means "not one," use a singular verb:

- None of the applicants for research grants is fully qualified.

In sentences with more than one subject, the linkage "neither…nor" may create a problem with respect to the verb form. The correct verb form depends on whether you link singular or plural nouns. If the nouns linked are singular *and* plural, the noun nearest the verb determines the verb form:

- Neither the physician nor the patient was informed of the drug used. (Both linked nouns are singular.)

  Neither the preliminary findings nor the final data were conclusive. (Both linked nouns are plural.)

  Neither the PhD supervisor nor his students were willing to contribute to the scientific meeting. (The noun closest to the verb is plural.)

4.5 Syntax (Order of Words)

4.5.1 Modifying Phrases

For a sentence to make sense, the words must be presented in a logical sequence. If the words are not in reasonable order, the result can be ridiculous, as shown below:

- *Confusing syntax*: We selected an investigator with considerable expertise in the field called Mike Miller.
  Confusing syntax: The study involved a small group of children in a Swiss children's hospital with juvenile diabetes.

Is the expertise called Mike Miller? Does the Swiss hospital suffer from juvenile diabetes? Clearly, the investigator was called Mike Miller, and the children suffered from juvenile diabetes. Because we frequently overlook faulty syntax and extract the intended message, such errors of syntax may go unnoticed by both the writer and the editor.

- *Clear syntax*: We selected an investigator called Mike Miller who has considerable expertise in the field.
  Clear syntax: The study involved a small group of children with juvenile diabetes in a Swiss children's hospital.

! Modifying phrases should be as close as possible to the words, phrases, or clauses they modify.

4.5.2 Position of Adverbs in Sentences

Adverbs qualify verbs, adjectives, or other adverbs. A traditional rule of grammar says that the adverb should *follow*, rather than split, the infinitive of the verb in sentences where the adverb modifies the verb. This issue has created much attention over the years. Even writers who know little about English grammar seem to be aware of the rule that infinitives (e.g., to go) should not be split by an adverb (e.g., to boldly go).

However, most grammarians and linguists will agree that this rule is no longer absolute, and that there are many situations in scientific writing where splitting the infinitive actually makes sense. Again, meaning is more important than rigid adherence to useless rules.

Let us consider some examples:

- *Grammatically correct*: It is the investigator's duty to inform the patient *fully* before initiating the therapy.
  Preferred because the meaning is clearer: It is the investigator's duty to *fully* inform the patient before initiating the therapy.

The first sentence is grammatically correct in that the infinitive (to inform) is left intact. In the second sentence, the adverb "fully" splits the infinitive but qualifies the nature of the information to be provided to the patient. Although we are breaking a rule of grammar, the second sentence simplifies the meaning and is therefore preferred.

Similarly, the adverb is sometimes best placed before the participle in passive sentences if special emphasis is required:

- *Grammatically correct*: The laboratory listings were screened *carefully* for any values above or below the defined normal ranges.
  Preferred because the meaning is clearer: The laboratory listings were *carefully* screened for any values above or below the defined normal ranges.

Table 4.10 shows other examples where placing the adverb before the verb makes sense.

Table 4.10 Placing the Adverb Before the Verb for Emphasis

GRAMMATICALLY CORRECT	PREFERRED BECAUSE OF SPECIAL EMPHASIS
The hypothesis was confirmed definitively in all instances.	The hypothesis was definitively confirmed in all instances.
Patients were allocated randomly to one of the three treatment groups.	Patients were randomly allocated to one of the three treatment groups.
The study was designed specifically to meet this goal.	The study was specifically designed to meet this goal.
The causative organism was identified unequivocally.	The causative organism was unequivocally identified.

> ! If the adverb strongly qualifies the verb, i.e., if you wish to place special emphasis on the nature of the action, it is legitimate to split the infinitive.

4.5.3 Position of Prepositions in Sentences

Most scientific communicators seem to know the rule that prepositions should not end a sentence. However, by rigidly adhering to this rule, writers run the risk of producing stilted, confusing messages. According to an old story, Winston Churchill once made this comment about a sentence that clumsily avoided a prepositional ending: "This is the sort of English up with which I will not put!" (In: Plain Words, by Sir Edwin Gowers, first published in 1948).

Most modern grammarians and linguists take a more open approach to this rule; some even go so far as to state that the rule should be done away with. (Note the preposition "with" at the end of the sentence!)

The following examples are grammatically correct, although the final word of the sentence happens to be a preposition:

> - You may question what this rule is for.
>   The patients were asked whether they found the diary easy to work with.
>   The effect of the ointment depended on the body part it was applied on.

Although prepositions at the end of a sentence are no longer an issue, we may still be on safer ground if syntax can be rearranged. Let us consider the following example:

> - *Acceptable but awkward*: Computer technology was the main subject he opted for.
>   *Preferable*: He opted for computer technology as his main subject.

Clearly, we shift the emphasis from "computer technology" in the first sentence to the person ("he") in the second. Often, the emphasis is intended, and in these cases you may end your sentence with a preposition if deemed appropriate.

> ! Although you may end a sentence with a preposition, place the preposition within the sentence if the same meaning is achieved.

4.6 Dangling Participles (and Other Danglers)

4.6.1 What Are Danglers?

Unfortunately, verbal phrase danglers are abundant in scientific reporting. They contribute substantially to misleading messages and confused writing. In most cases, the problem arises from a lack of logical thinking or poor word order. Many danglers escape the author's and/or editor's attention because the readers' brains may deduce the intended message, disregarding the fact that the sentence says something totally different. Needless to say, guesswork is incompatible with science, and it is unacceptable to let our readers guess what we have meant to say.

4.6.2 Dangling Participles

A participle is a verb form that acts as an adjective. Most participles end in "ing," "ed," or "en." Participles have some of the features of a verb, such as tense, voice, and requirement for an object.

A participle is said to "dangle" if its implied subject is not the subject of the main clause of the sentence. Thus, a dangling participle implies an actor but does not specify who or what it is, thereby leaving proper participle–subject matching up to the reader. In some instances, this may lead to gross misinterpretations.

Let us consider an example:

- *Incorrect because of dangling participle*: Structured into various sections, the readers of this review can choose the topic of primary interest.

Here, the participle ("structured") appears to refer to the readers. Clearly, it is the review that is structured into various sections. The author leaves this deduction to the reader. The sentence can be corrected as follows:

- *Correct*: The review is structured into various sections, which allows the readers to choose the topic of primary interest.

Similarly, participles ending in "ing" often cause danglers in scientific writing:

- *Incorrect because of dangling participle*: Paying attention to the rules of good writing, most texts can be improved.

It is not the texts that should pay attention to the rules; it is the writers. To correct the sentence, remove the dangling participle:

- *Correct*: Most texts can be improved if writers pay attention to the rules of good writing.

One participle that often causes problems is "based on." Let us look at an example:

- *Incorrect because of dangling participle*: Based on experience, microsomal preparations are more useful than hepatocytes.

Are microsomal preparations based on experience? Clearly, the authors base their conclusion on experience. You can untangle the sentence by either making "experience" the subject of the sentence or using the personal pronoun "we":

- *Correct*: Experience shows that microsomal preparations are more useful than hepatocytes.

    Better because active: We consider microsomal preparations more useful than hepatocytes.

The two "-ing" words "following" and "using" are particularly troublesome. Thus, it is good advice to avoid them wherever possible, as shown in Table 4.11.

Table 4.11 Avoiding "Following" and "Using"

AVOID	PREFERRED
Following the appropriate guidelines, the abstracts were much clearer.	*The abstracts were much clearer if authors followed (or applied) the appropriate guidelines.*
Using a validated HPLC method, four metabolites were detected.	*Four metabolites were detected by a validated HPLC method.* Better because active: *We detected four metabolites by the use of a validated HPLC method.*

! Carefully check proper participle–subject matching in sentences that include a participle.

4.6.3 Dangling Gerunds

Not all "-ing" words are participles. Gerunds also end in "ing," but they act as nouns rather than as adjectives. Like dangling participles, dangling gerunds imply an actor without specifying the person or thing.

> ● *Incorrect because of dangling gerund*: After terminating drug treatment, behavioral therapy is recommended.
>
> *Better*: Behavioral therapy is recommended after discontinuation of drug treatment.

The upper sentence implies that behavioral therapy terminates drug treatment. Again, the actor, i.e., the person stopping the therapy, is just assumed but not specified.

> ! Avoid dangling gerunds by using an alternative noun and proper word order.

> Exercise 7

4.7 The Relative Pronouns "Which" and "That"

Proper usage of "that" and "which" troubles many writers, as does the question whether or not a comma should be placed before these pronouns. Relative pronouns refer to a previous noun in subordinate clauses. The pronoun "that" introduces a restrictive clause, i.e., a clause that is essential to the meaning of the sentence. In such sentences, there is no comma before the relative pronoun. In the past, the only possible pronoun in such sentences was "that," but nowadays many writers use "which" in place of "that." In principle, this is permissible as long as the comma is omitted if "which" introduces a restrictive clause.

Below are two examples of correct usage of "that" and "which" in restrictive clauses.

> ● The books that (or which) provide exercises are particularly helpful.
>
> The substances which (or that) performed best in the screening test were those that had a simple chemical structure.

In contrast to the restrictive clause, the nonrestrictive clause is not essential to the meaning of the sentence; it merely provides some additional information. Here, the relative pronoun is always "which" and must be preceded by a comma.

Let us consider these examples:

- Some books provide exercises, which is particularly helpful.

    The substances with a simple chemical structure performed best in the screening test, which was an unexpected finding.

In essence, "which" that replaces "that" always introduces a restrictive clause supplying essential information. In these sentences, a comma before "which" (or "that") is incorrect. However, if "which" introduces a nonrestrictive clause supplying only incidental or additional information, a comma before "which" is mandatory.

4.8 Use of "Respectively"

In scientific literature, few words cause more confusion than the term "respectively." Scientific writers of German tongue often use the term in place of the German word "respektive." In English, "respektive" is usually a simple "or," and overabundant use of "respectively" frequently obscures the issue.

- *Incorrect*: We used TLC and HPLC, respectively, for analyzing the samples.
    Correct: We used TLC or HPLC for analyzing the samples.

The word "respectively" indicates a one-to-one correspondence that may not otherwise be apparent between items of two series. If only one series is listed, then the use of "respectively" is incorrect.

- *Incorrect*: Incubation times were 2 h, 6 h, and 12 h, respectively.
    Correct: Incubation times for experiments 1, 2, and 3 were 2 h, 6 h, and 12 h, respectively.

Confusing sentences containing "respectively" can often be reworded to avoid this troublesome word:

- *Correct but cumbersome*: Adverse event rates for the low dose and high dose were below 10% and 20%, respectively.
  Better: Adverse event rates were below 10% for the low dose and below 20% for the high dose.

! Only use "respectively" if two series are listed and if there could be ambiguity. Use a comma before "respectively."

> Exercise 8

4.9 Plurals of Abstractions and Attributes

Plurals of abstractions and attributes often cause difficulty in scientific writing. Let us consider an example:

- The mood of the child changed suddenly.

In the sentence above, would three children have three moods? Although it may seem logical to use the plural if you refer to more than one individual abstractions (e.g., behavior, mood, curiosity, or emotion) or attributes possessed in common (e.g., tolerability, efficacy, or effectiveness) are used in the singular.

- *Incorrect*: The stimulant drug clearly affected the behaviors of the mice.
  Correct: The stimulant drug clearly affected the behavior of the mice.

  Incorrect: The treatments achieved marked efficacies in all patients.
  Correct: The treatments achieved marked efficacy in all patients.

! Use the singular for abstractions and attributes possessed in common.

Putting It Nicely: Style   5

> *"The administrator with a sense for style hates waste;*
> *the engineer with a sense for style economizes his material;*
> *the artisan with a sense for style prefers good work.*
> *Style is the ultimate morality of mind."*
>
> Alfred North Whitehead

5.1 What Is "Style" in the Context of Scientific Writing?

"Style" is one of those terms that can mean anything or nothing at all. Robert Day defines "style" as the "personality" of a scientific manuscript (see Robert Day 2011). He emphasizes that each publication has its own "personality," dictated by both the writing style used and the particular journal's editorial requirements.

Good scientific writing is not only a matter of correctness; it is often just as much a question of good style and careful adherence to stylistic conventions used in a particular field of science. Many competent scientists hold the firm belief that style is just "nice to have" without lending any importance to the scientific message. Let me assure you that no one charged with the difficult task of editing and proofreading manuscripts would share this view. A clear and consistent writing style not only facilitates the "digestion" of the scientific message; it also shortens the time-consuming process of editing and helps to make the task enjoyable.

In this chapter, I draw your attention to stylistic issues that are not necessarily a question of "right" or "wrong" but clearly enhance the readability and clarity of your text. In particular, this chapter deals with the issue of active versus passive voice, the need to reduce the number of prepositions, and the sensible handling of modifiers and other "decorative" words in scientific texts. Moreover, we shall look at journal-specific style recommendations, i.e., the so-called house styles, and company-internal conventions of style and format.

5.2 Active Versus Passive Voice

5.2.1 Why Argue About Active/Passive Voice?

Passive versus active voice in scientific writing has been a controversial issue for many years. Without any doubt, the tradition of using the passive voice in scientific reporting is firmly engraved in scientists' brains. Many scientific communicators believe that it is inappropriate, even impolite, to use personal pronouns, such as "I" or "we." They would prefer to say, "it was studied" rather than "I studied" or "we studied." Note here that the passive sentence does not tell us who studied the subject in question. In his book published in 1971, John Swales states that "… *passive sentences are clearer. The first reason for this is that passive sentences do not mention people. For a scientist, many references to people are unnecessary and confusing.*"

Nowadays, most modern grammarians, linguists, and editors agree that the exclusive use of the passive voice is redundant. In this time and age where brevity and conciseness critically impact on review and approval of a manuscript, the active voice helps to keep messages lean and clear. Moreover, our time constraints with both the writing and reading of scientific information call for an unambiguous language involving active verbs and personal pronouns wherever possible.

5.2.2 Shifting Emphasis by Choosing the Voice

If the subject of the sentence performs the action, the sentence is in the active voice, but if the subject of the sentence is the recipient of the action, the sentence is passive.

> ● *Active*: The team studied the genetic mutations.
> *Passive*: The genetic mutations were studied by the team.

Although the two sentences say more or less the same thing, the emphasis is different. While the active sentence stresses the "doer," i.e., the team, the passive wording places emphasis on the subject studied, i.e., the genetic mutations. You may argue that the voice makes little difference to the overall statement, but you will notice that the passive sentence uses more words than the active sentence.

There are two ways to make a sentence active, namely by using a subject (such as "team" in the sentence above) plus an active verb (e.g., "studied") or by using personal pronouns (e.g., "we"). Although the active voice should be our first choice, the exclusive use of active sentences is sometimes inappropriate and often impossible. Thus, we have to find our own "healthy" ratio of passive versus active formulations.

Here is a useful rule to remember:

> ! Use the active voice most of the time because it is more direct and less wordy. If you want to emphasize the action rather than the agent, use the passive voice, bearing in mind that the proportion of passive verbs should not exceed 30%.

5.2.3 The Verb "To Be" in Copula Formulations

One of the arguments in favor of active-voice sentences concerns the abundance of the verb "to be" in scientific literature. "To be" does not only occur in every passive sentence but may also be used in so-called copula formulations where the verb links the subject with its complement. Here, "to be" acts as the main verb in sentences that do not describe any action. Although such constructions are not strictly passive, they add to the tiresome abundance of sentences containing the verb "to be." Here are some examples of such sentences:

> ● Dr Sarah Craven is the author of the book.
> The design of the clinical trial was deficient.
> The batch numbers were the same in all cases.
> Hydrolysis of the prodrug in human intestinal tissue was rapid.

> ! Copula formulations are frequently essential. However, a powerful alternative for the verb "to be" may sometimes make the sentence more interesting.

> > Exercise 9

5.3 Overuse of Prepositions

Winston Churchill once described prepositions as an enormously versatile part of grammar, as in "*What made you pick this book I didn't want to be read to out of up for?*" I guess it takes a special talent to construct a sentence that ends with five prepositions in a row. At the same time, it takes a special skill to grasp such messages on first reading.

Prepositions are connecting links showing a relationship between the object of the preposition and the modifying prepositional sentence. Therefore, clear communication would not be possible without prepositions, but scientific writers often use them too liberally because rewording of the sentence would mean a special effort. In fact, many a writing expert would insist that the overuse of prepositions in scientific writing is the single most important cause of confused messages.

There are approximately 70 prepositions in the English language. They can be broadly classified as prepositions of time and date, movement, location, or limitation, as shown in Table 5.1.

Table 5.1 Types of Prepositions

TYPES OF PREPOSITIONS	EXAMPLES
Time / date	*at, by, on, before, in, from, since, for, during, to, until, after*
Movement	*from, to, at, in, by, into, onto, off, out, out of, over, under*
Location	*in, above, over, under, below, beneath, underneath, between, behind, among, with*
Limitation	*but, except, without*

We all have seen (if not written) sentences like this one:

> ● *Abundant prepositions*: The data **from** the participants **of** younger age **in** this study were compared **with** those **of** subjects **of** older age **by** an analysis **of** variance.

This sentence consists of 25 words, 8 of which are prepositions. In other words, almost every third word is a preposition, and this is clearly too many. A "rule of thumb" is to use less than one preposition in every four words. Consider this correction of the above sentence:

> ● *"Healthy" ratio of prepositions*: The data **from** the younger and older study participants were compared **by** an analysis **of** variance.

The sentence now contains 16 words, 3 of which are prepositions. Thus, the ratio of prepositions to other words is <1:5. Because the "of" in "analysis of variance" is part of a fixed term, this preposition must be retained.

Of course, we could improve the style of the above sentence even further by using the active voice, as long as we were the agents, that is, the "doers," in this case:

> ● *Preferred because active*: We compared the data from the younger and older study participants by an analysis of variance.

Table 5.2 shows some rules whose application will help to limit the number of prepositions in scientific texts.

5.4 Limiting Modifiers and Other Decorative Words

Table 5.2 Rules for Limiting Prepositions

RULES	EXAMPLES
Delete an entire prepositional phrase as meaningless or unnecessary.	In order to confirm the data.... Better: To confirm the data ...
Convert a prepositional phrase into a participle.	In the attempt to demonstrate this effect in vitro, ... Better: Attempting to demonstrate this effect in vitro, ...
Convert a prepositional phrase into an adverb.	Of the data sets tested by statistics, three were significant. Better: Of the data sets tested statistically, three were significant. Better still: Three data sets were statistically significant.
Change passive voice to active voice.	The hematocrit was determined by the nurse. Better: The nurse determined the hematocrit.
Split long sentences.	In our study, we found a positive correlation between the subjects' brain activity (as measured by EEG) and their subjective sensation of stimulation, and this finding was consistent across all subjects tested. Better: In our study, we found a positive correlation between the subjects' brain activity (as measured by EEG) and their subjective sensation of stimulation. This finding was ...

! Use prepositions in a "healthy" proportion to the remaining words of the sentence (i.e., no more than one preposition per four words).

> Exercise 10

5.4 Limiting Modifiers and Other Decorative Words

5.4.1 Excessive Adjectives, Adverbs, and Nouns

Modifiers specify or describe the meaning of another term. In most cases, modifiers are adjectives (modifying nouns), adverbs (modifying verbs, adjectives, or other adverbs), or nouns (modifying other nouns). Table 5.3 shows examples of each modifier type.

Table 5.3 Examples of Modifiers

TYPES OF MODIFIERS	EXAMPLES
Adjective	*a* reproducible *assay* *a* large *patient population* positive *serum samples*
Adverb	*the* deeply *colored stain* *a* very *successful experiment* *a* statistically significantly *higher result*
Noun	enzyme *immunoassay* tissue *factor* regression *line*

Modifiers add richness, sparkle, and precision to otherwise dull descriptions, but overloading scientific statements with unnecessary decorative words distracts the reader. The verbosity frequently encountered in scientific literature is often the result of too many modifiers that do not add information but rather obscure the actual message. Let us consider an example:

> ● *Excessive use of modifiers*: These impressive as well as clinically and statistically significant data are of great and unique importance to this rather poorly researched field of neurobiological science and will substantially add to the presently still modest knowledge of cognitive processing in the elderly.

What did the author try to tell us? Surely, we would have less trouble to understand the message had the author used fewer modifiers:

> ● *Fewer modifiers*: These statistically significant data substantially add to the current understanding of cognitive processing in the elderly.

The example above illustrates that overloading a text with modifiers renders the writing flabby and ungraceful. Thus, a good approach is to use only those adjectives, adverbs, and noun modifiers necessary to qualify the intended statement. As Mark Twain put it: "*As to the adjective, when in doubt, strike it out.*"

> ! Use modifiers in moderation. Limit the number of decorative words to those that add necessary information to the statement.

5.4.2 Modifier Strings

Some languages, German for example, permit the use of modifier clusters to describe another word, usually a noun. English is more ruthless with modifier strings. Usually, two descriptive words that qualify another term are about as far as you can go. Take a look at this muddled sentence:

> ● *Modifier strings in sentences*: The blinded report procedure planning meeting organization was done by the clinical trial monitor.

This awkward sentence can only be cured of its modifier strings by replacing some nouns with verbs:

- *Acceptable use of modifiers*: The clinical trial monitor organized the meeting to plan the blinded report procedure.

Unfortunately, there are many officially used names of organizations, committees, procedures, databases, or illnesses that clearly violate the rule stated above. In these situations, we are not usually at liberty to change the strings. Here are some examples:

- *Modifier strings in names*: Peer Review Congress Advisory Board, Clinical Research and Development Decision-Making Steps and Procedures, Drug Safety and Efficacy Advisory Committee

! Avoid modifier strings in sentences, names, and titles.

> Exercise 11

5.5 The "House Style" of Journals

Nowadays, most good journals provide detailed instructions for authors of manuscripts seeking publication. Such instructions are commonly referred to as the journal's "house style." Although individual house styles may still vary to some extent, considerable effort has gone into harmonizing standards and formats among scientific journals. The most important initiative in this respect is the generation of the document entitled *Uniform Requirements for Manuscripts Submitted to Biomedical Journals: Writing and Editing for Biomedical Publication* (current version available from http://www.icmje.org). For further information on the background, purpose, and impact of this document, see Sect. 7.2.

Hundreds of biomedical journals have agreed to use the *Uniform Requirements*. These journals are encouraged to state in the instructions for authors that their requirements are in accordance with the current version of the guideline. Authors will find it helpful to follow the recommendations in this document whenever possible. Adherence to this guideline improves the quality and clarity of manuscripts submitted to any journal, as well as the ease of editing.

At the same time, every journal has editorial requirements uniquely suited to its purposes. Therefore, authors should familiarize themselves with the specific instructions for authors and should apply them consistently. The Mulford Library at the Medical College of Ohio maintains a useful compendium of instructions for authors (available from http://mulford.meduohio.edu).

When scrutinizing the various instructions for authors, you will find that the level of detail varies considerably among the journals. While many of the principles of individual house styles are standards of good writing and proper use of grammar, some requirements appear to be fairly arbitrary. Why would one journal prefer British spelling and another American spelling? I would argue that even the arbitrary style recommendations make sense in an effort to maintain consistency of papers within any particular journal. It is for this reason that certain house styles have become readily recognized as a particular journal's hallmark. Good examples are *The Lancet* and the *British Medical Journal* (*BMJ*), whose style recommendations extend far beyond the preparation of a manuscript (current versions available from http://www.thelancet.com/for-authors and http://www.bmj.com/about-bmj/resources-authors, respectively).

With the aim to promote clarity of thought and expression, a good house style embraces the use of first-person pronouns, the active voice of verbs, and short sentences. At the same time, good guidelines are ruthless with noun clusters and other unnecessary modifier strings, dangling participles, tautologies, and the many misuses of punctuation. In addition, the journal's house style imposes technical accuracy in tables, figures, and other data displays or use of drug names.

> ! Before drafting a manuscript, consult the current version of the *Uniform Requirements* as well as the specific instructions for authors of the selected journal.

5.6 Company-Internal Conventions of Style and Format

Although much effort has gone into harmonizing style conventions for international exchange of scientific information, some organizations maintain a tradition of casual reporting. The tradition of poor writing is often handed down from supervisors to staff members, who, in turn, pass it on to new employees with limited writing experience. In my workshops, I frequently challenge certain "inbred" conventions, to which I usually get the reply: "We have always done it this way!"

Serious deficiencies in the reporting of scientific data usually become apparent only when documents are submitted to health authorities (in the process of obtaining authorization for marketing of a new product) or journal editors (when intending to publish data). These official institutions impose strict requirements on the clarity and accuracy of the scientific message. The most frequent deficiencies are these:
- poorly designed templates for preclinical, clinical, and technical documents
- jargonized writing and use of "inbred" terms with uncertain meaning
- mixing of British and American spelling within and across documents
- modifier strings and misuse of adjectives and adverbs
- exclusive use of the passive voice to avoid the naming of responsible persons

5.6 Company-Internal Conventions of Style and Format

- erroneous use of punctuation, especially commas, brackets, parentheses, and semicolons
- inconsistent use of capitals in titles, drug names, departments, etc.

> ! Poor writing style handed down by tradition will delay review of the document. This, in turn, prolongs the "time to market" of publications and applications for marketing authorization of new drugs. An internal style manual to be used by all contributors can be a great help.

Redundancy and Jargon: Focusing on the Essentials

6

"Most of the fundamental ideas of science are essentially simple, and may, as a rule, be expressed in a language comprehensible to everyone."

Albert Einstein

6.1 Redundancies in Scientific Reporting

Redundancies are common troublemakers in scientific communication. They come in various forms, some more obvious than others, but all of them unnecessary or even disturbing. Common redundancies include double negatives or doubling of words that have the same meaning (tautology).

Many of the words or expressions we use in scientific writing are useless, but we still go on using them, mostly because others do so, too. When I mention such terms in my lectures, students often argue that they have seen the term in print, which they regard as proof of validity. My answer to this is that many useless or even incorrect terms or expressions have been published and are being published, but this does not necessarily make them "correct."

It is true that traditions tend to change over time. A previously incorrect term may gradually become accepted because of its broad exposure. An example that springs to mind is "tolerance," a French word that has found its way into English usage in clinical reporting over the years. Another term illustrating the evolutionary nature of scientific English is "data." This plural form of the singular "datum" is being increasingly used as a collective noun, i.e., a noun that is plural in meaning but singular in form (see also Sect. 4.4.3). Thus, many writers prefer to say, "this data shows," although the plural would be grammatically correct (i.e., these data show). Personally, I still favor proper subject–verb matching in this case, although I accept that "data" may eventually be declared a collective noun.

While the terms discussed above deserve your critical eye, there are many expressions that should simply be avoided. In the following, we will consider some typical causes of redundant and jargonized writing.

6.2 Double Negatives

Double negatives are rarely needed in scientific reporting. More often than not, they render statements clumsy and difficult to grasp. A second negative usually cancels the first. Table 6.1 lists some common double negatives and offers a positive alternative.

Table 6.1 Double Negatives and Their Positive Meaning

CONFUSING DOUBLE NEGATIVES	PREFERABLE (POSITIVE STATEMENT)
Diabetes is not uncommon among hypertensive patients.	*Diabetes is common among hypertensive patients.*
Not very many of the laboratory tests were negative.	*Most laboratory tests were positive.*
Nausea and vomiting were not infrequently reported during the treatment phase.	*Nausea and vomiting were frequently reported during the treatment phase.*
Although the DNA sequencing was not unsuccessful, we decided to repeat it.	*Although the DNA sequencing was successful, we decided to repeat it.*
It is not unusual for scientists to hypothesize too readily.	*Scientists tend to hypothesize too readily.*

! If the statement is positive, state it in the positive.

6.3 Tautology (Repeated and Redundant Words)

Tautology is the repetition of words with similar meaning, often disguised and always undetected by the spell checker. Avoiding tautologies is an important measure to keep scientific texts as lean as possible. Moreover, needless repetition of the same message in different words confuses the reader.

Table 6.2 shows some typical examples of tautological and otherwise redundant expressions. Section 11.4 lists other awkward phrases to avoid.

Table 6.2 Tautological and Redundant Expressions to Avoid

TAUTOLOGY	PREFERRED TERM
adequate enough	*adequate* (*or enough*)
advance planning	*planning*
appear(s) to be	*appear(s)*
approximately 1000 to 1200	*approximately 1100*
basic essentials	*basics* (*or essentials*)
basic fundamentals	*basics* (*or fundamentals*)
close proximity	*proximity*
consensus of opinion	*consensus*
cooperated together	*cooperated*
definite decision	*decision*
elongate in length	*elongate*
extremely minimal	*minimal*
first priority	*priority*
future predictions	*predictions*
green colored	*green*
increase in increments	*increase*
initial prototype (model)	*prototype*
intradermal skin injection	*intradermal injection*
joint cooperation	*cooperation*
major breakthrough	*breakthrough*
modern science of today	*modern science*
most optimum	*optimum*
necessary requirement	*requirement*
outside periphery	*periphery*
past history	*past* (*or history*)
rate of speed	*speed*
resemble in appearance	*resemble*
true facts	*facts*
twelve in number	*twelve*
usual rule	*rule*
very unique	*unique*

! Do not duplicate terms and expressions.

6.4 Doubling Prepositions

Clumsy writing may sometimes come from the doubling of prepositions, as shown in the examples below:

> ● *Incorrect*: I cannot comment on the importance of this finding because the topic is **outside of** my own field.
> *Correct*: I cannot comment on the importance of this finding because the topic is **outside** my own field.

> ● *Incorrect*: The test mice remained **inside of** their cages during the entire experimental period.
> *Correct*: The test mice remained **inside** their cages during the entire experimental period.

"Inside" and "outside" are prepositions, as is "of." Other prepositions often leading to erroneous doubling are "between" (as in "in between"), "except" (as in "except of"), or "above" and "below."

6.5 Jargonized Writing

Scientific groups often use their own jargons that may well be understood by the members of such groups. However, authors are often unaware that no one outside their group uses these terms. This applies just as much to abbreviations and acronyms that are not commonly understood.

Let us consider an example:

> ● Values of CV varied considerably.

What does CV stand for? The abbreviation can mean several different things, such as cardiovascular, coefficient of variation, or even curriculum vitae.

If you have the slightest doubt as to whether an abbreviation is commonly accepted, avoid the expression or use the full term instead. It may be helpful to consult the international scientific literature when trying to establish whether the scientific community uses a certain term or not.

In clinical reporting, we tend to find some typical errors that come about by using jargons, careless language, or simply an inappropriate term. Table 6.3 shows some examples.

Table 6.3 Typical Clinical Jargons and Other Examples of Careless Writing

JARGON OR CARELESS WRITING	CORRECT
The patient was discontinued because of an adverse event.	The patient was withdrawn from the study because of an adverse event. Or (better because active voice): The patient discontinued the study because of an adverse event.
The patient was randomized to receive a dose of 10 mg/kg.	The patient was randomly allocated to a dose of 10 mg/kg. Or: The patient was allocated at random to a dose of 10 mg/kg.
Local tolerance of the topical antifungal cream was poor.	Local tolerability of the topical antifungal cream was poor.
By the time he was admitted, his rapid heart had stopped, and he was feeling better.	By the time he was admitted, his heartbeat had slowed, and he was feeling better.
She left her red blood cells at another hospital.	She left the records of her red blood cell counts at another hospital.
Effectiveness and tolerance of the 5% ibuprofen gel were assessed on 20 healthy volunteers in this study.	This study assessed the efficacy and tolerability of the 5% ibuprofen gel in 20 healthy volunteers.
The difference between the two dose groups was statistically insignificant.	The difference between the two dose groups was not statistically significant.
The recommended dosage was 500 mg.	The recommended dose was 500 mg. Or: The recommended dosage was 500 mg once daily.

! Resist the temptation to use jargon in scientific writing. Always apply your common sense before adopting a term from others.

6.6 Oxymorons

Oxymorons are contradictory expressions. How can terms such as "false facts" or a "genuine lie" make sense? Because oxymorons tend to be ambivalent, they should be avoided in scientific writing. Nonetheless, there are a few oxymorons that are commonly used. Examples are ill health, common sense, bad grammar, disorganized system, conspicuous absences, or cruel kindness.

! When using an oxymoron, make sure the term is commonly known and its use is appropriate in scientific communication.

> Exercise 12

Quoting Published Material: Reference Formats

> "Great discoveries and improvements invariably
> involve the cooperation of many minds.
> I may be given credit for having blazed the trail,
> but when I look at the subsequent developments
> I feel the credit is due to others
> rather than to myself."
>
> Alexander Graham Bell

7.1 What Can Go Wrong When Quoting Published Material?

References in reports and journal articles serve two main purposes, namely documentation and acknowledgment. In either case, references form a critical part of the manuscript and must therefore undergo close scrutiny by both the author(s) and editor(s). Studies show that 50% to 70% of all quoted literature references contain at least one erroneous item. These errors come about by copying lists of references from previous papers or reports that are likely to contain irregularities. In this way, mistakes are carried over, and verification of the original information becomes difficult. Common deficiencies range from simple typing errors to gross misquoting of titles or author names.

When quoting published material, do not copy down references from citations or databases, however credible, since these usually pay insufficient attention to detail and often contain erroneous author initials, page numbers, or even years of publication. Thus, the only reliable source is the original paper as published in its original journal.

Do bear in mind that any mistake in quoting references will make it difficult to trace the original article, and precious time to completing the manuscript or report will be lost. It is for this reason that authors must pay utmost attention to the exact wording and format of quoted literature references.

7.2 Reference Formats and the Uniform Requirements

7.2.1 What Style Should I Use?

Styles of handling references vary considerably, and many different formats exist. Some companies create their own internal conventions that may deviate from commonly used journal styles (see also Sect. 5.6). Whatever reference style is followed, consistency throughout the manuscript (report, journal article, or book) is important.

An effort has been made to harmonize reference formats across journals and other documents to minimize citation errors and facilitate retrieval of quoted material. A small group of editors of general medical journals met informally in 1978 in Vancouver, British Columbia, to establish guidelines for the format of manuscripts submitted to their journals. The group became known as the Vancouver Group. Their requirements for manuscripts, including formats for bibliographic references developed by the National Library of Medicine (NLM), were first published in 1979.

Subsequently, the Vancouver Group expanded and evolved into the International Committee of Medical Journal Editors (ICMJE) which meets annually. The ICMJE has gradually broadened its concerns to include other aspects of scientific reporting, e.g., ethical principles related to publication in biomedical journals. Meanwhile, the ICMJE has produced multiple editions of the *Uniform Requirements for Manuscripts Submitted to Biomedical Journals*, and the guideline is updated regularly. When consulting this important document, please use the current version (available from http://www.icmje.org).

7.2.2 Using Vancouver Style

The *Uniform Requirements* suggest the bibliographic style formats that were developed for uniformity by the NLM. Because of its origin, this reference style is termed Vancouver style. Since Vancouver style continues to gain broad acceptance, this format is almost always the bibliographic style of choice (see also Sect. 5.5).

Unless the journal specifies a different convention, references should be numbered consecutively in the order in which they are first mentioned in the text. Identify references in text, tables, and legends by Arabic numerals in parentheses. The titles of journals should be abbreviated according to the style used in *Index Medicus*. Consult the *List of Journals Indexed in Index Medicus* published annually as a separate publication by the library and as a list in the January issue of *Index Medicus*. The list can also be obtained through the library's website (http://www.nlm.nih.gov).

For standard journal articles, list all authors if there are six or fewer. For more than six authors, list the first six, followed by et al. (Please note that most examples cited below were taken from the current version of the *Uniform Requirements for Manuscripts Submitted to Biomedical Journals*.)

7.2 Reference Formats and the Uniform Requirements

> ● Fette A, Mayr J. Slipped distal humerus epiphysis in tiny infants easily detected and followed up by ultrasound. Ultraschall Med. 2012 Dec;33(7):361–363.
>
> Rose ME, Huerbin MB, Melick J, Marion DW, Palmer AM, Schiding JK, et al. Regulation of interstitial excitatory amino acid concentrations after cortical contusion injury. Brain Res. 2002;935(1-2):40–46.

As an option, the month and issue number may be omitted if a journal carries continuous pagination throughout a volume (as many medical journals do):

> ● Fette A, Mayr J. Slipped distal humerus epiphysis in tiny infants easily detected and followed up by ultrasound. Ultraschall Med. 2012;33:361–363.

If no author is given, state the title and journal details as follows:

> ● 21st century heart solution may have a sting in the tail. BMJ. 2002;325(7357):184.

For volumes or issues with supplements, state "suppl" where appropriate:

> ● Geraud G, Spierings EL, Keywood C. Tolerability and safety of frovatriptan with short- and long-term use for treatment of migraine and in comparison with sumatriptan. Headache. 2002;42 Suppl 2:S93–S99.
>
> Glauser TA. Integrating clinical trial data into clinical practice. Neurology. 2002;58(12 Suppl 7):S6-S12.

Consult the current version of the *Uniform Requirements for Manuscripts Submitted to Biomedical Journals* (available from http://www.icmje.org) for more details, e.g., for references without issue or volume, or for articles containing retraction.

The style used for citing books depends on whether personal author(s) or editor(s) as authors are given:

> ● Murray PR, Rosenthal KS, Kobayashi GS, Pfaller MA. Medical microbiology. 4th ed. St. Louis: Mosby; 2002.
>
> Gilstrap LC 3rd, Cunningham FG, VanDorsten JP, editors. Operative obstetrics. 2nd ed. New York: McGraw-Hill; 2002.

The format used for chapters in a book is as follows:

> • Meltzer PS, Kallioniemi A, Trent JM. Chromosome alterations in human solid tumors. In: Vogelstein B, Kinzler KW, editors. The genetic basis of human cancer. New York: McGraw-Hill; 2002. p. 93–113.

Conference proceedings and conference papers often cause difficulties. Examples are shown below:

> • Harnden P, Joffe JK, Jones WG, editors. Germ cell tumours V. Proceedings of the 5th Germ Cell Tumour Conference; 2001 Sep 13–15; Leeds, UK. New York: Springer; 2002.
>
> Christensen S, Oppacher F. An analysis of Koza's computational effort statistic for genetic programming. In: Foster JA, Lutton E, Miller J, Ryan C, Tettamanzi AG, editors. Genetic programming. EuroGP 2002: Proceedings of the 5th European Conference on Genetic Programming; 2002 Apr 3–5; Kinsdale, Ireland. Berlin: Springer; 2002. p. 182–91.

For details on how to quote a scientific or technical report, dissertation, or patent, consult the current version of the *Uniform Requirements for Manuscripts Submitted to Biomedical Journals* (http://www.icmje.org). The guidelines also provide information on citing other published material, such as dictionaries, newspaper articles, audiovisual material, or legal material.

Avoid citing abstracts or personal communications unless they provide essential information not available from a public source. In this case, the name of the person and date of communication should be cited in parentheses in the text. For scientific articles, authors should obtain written permission and confirmation of accuracy from the source of a personal communication.

Special attention should be paid to the citation of unpublished material. Unpublished material may include abstracts or articles presented at a society meeting (oral presentation or poster presentation) as well as material accepted for publication but not yet published.

Information from manuscripts submitted but not accepted should be cited in the text as "unpublished observations" with written permission from the source. For references to material accepted for publication but not yet published, the journal title is followed by "in press" or "forthcoming," depending on the journal's house style. (Note: NLM prefers "forthcoming" because not all items will be printed.)

Authors should obtain written permission to cite such papers as well as verification that the manuscript has been accepted for publication:

> ● Tian D, Araki H, Stahl E, Bergelson J, Kreitman M. Signature of balancing selection in Arabidopsis. Proc Natl Acad Sci U S A. Forthcoming 2002.

With the increased exchange of electronic material and the broad acceptance of such information, you can use online designation of articles or other published information if appropriate:

> ● Abood S. Quality improvement initiative in nursing homes: the ANA acts in an advisory role. Am J Nurs [Internet]. 2002 Jun [cited 2002 Aug 12];102(6):[about 1 p.]. Available from: http://www.nursingworld.org/AJN/2002/june/Wawatch.htm

If you cite programs or computer files, the nature of such material should be indicated in square brackets:

> ● Anderson SC, Poulsen KB. Anderson's electronic atlas of hematology [CD-ROM]. Philadelphia: Lippincott Williams & Wilkins; 2002.

> ! When quoting published or unpublished information, consult the journal's house style and follow the reference style consistently. If no specific guidelines are given, use Vancouver style.

7.2.3 Reference Manager Tools

Nowadays, many authors use a reference manager software to facilitate the formatting of reference lists. Such tools provide the formats for many of the standard reference styles accepted by journals. At the touch of a key, the entire reference list is formatted in a selected style. If your manuscript is rejected by the chosen journal, you can reformat the references to meet the requirements of another journal.

Reference manager tools are very accurate and tend to facilitate the handling of references, but authors must invest the time needed to get familiarized with the program. Moreover, editors and proofreaders must use the same reference manager tools if they wish to make changes to the manuscript.

Ethics of Scientific Writing: Avoiding Discrimination

8

> "Replacing sexist words and phrases with terms that treat all
> people respectfully can be satisfying and rewarding.
> It can also be difficult and frustrating,
> and it is good to admit that."
>
> Rosalie Maggio

8.1 Prejudice and Semantic Labeling

In recent years, writers, especially scientific writers, have become increasingly aware of language sensitivities. It is in the interest of the author to encourage the reader to carry on reading the manuscript or publication; thus, any offense to the reader will probably get in the way of this objective.

Readers may be upset by any term that excludes, embarrasses, hurts, or "labels" them. Such terms may be "sexist" or "racist" in nature, but it is fair to say that they are mostly used unconsciously and unintentionally. For this reason, it is essential that writers become sensitized to those terms and expressions that are likely to annoy, if not upset, the reader.

8.2 Sexist Writing and Gender-Biased Expressions

8.2.1 Sex Versus Gender

When do we use the term "sex," and when is "gender" appropriate? The question is a frequent one and cannot be settled easily in all cases. The *American Medical Association Manual of Style* has to say this:

"*Sex* refers to the biological characteristics of males and females. *Gender* includes more than sex and serves as a cultural indicator of a person's personal and social status. An important consideration when referring to sex is the level of specificity required: specify sex when it is relevant."

All very nice, but where does this leave us? Although I personally prefer the term "gender" as it is more neutral, the term "sex" is usually needed in demographic summaries or statistical outputs. This makes sense because the differences usually looked at in studies tend to be just the biological ones, disregarding social and personal status as they are irrelevant here.

8.2.2 Gender-Inclusive Language

Although sexist writing is no longer as common as it used to be, we still see too much of it in scientific texts. The problem arises because English has no singular pronoun that includes both males and females. Consequently, certain groups of people, such as patients, teachers, or medical professionals, are sometimes described as being exclusively male or female, as shown in the examples below:

> ● *Sexist writing*: The general practitioner should refer *his* patients to a specialist if he deems this necessary.
>
> *Sexist writing*: A study nurse will determine your blood pressure before and after the infusion. *She* will inform the study director of any abnormalities.

Clearly, a general practitioner may well be a woman, and the study nurse could just as well be a man. In the first sentence, sexist writing can be avoided if we use the plural:

> ● *Gender neutral*: General practitioners should refer *their* patients to a specialist if deemed necessary.

In the second sentence, the plural ("they") would not be appropriate since a single nurse is responsible for blood-pressure determinations. Here, we can be gender neutral only by using the unpopular "he/she" construction. Although many books on scientific writing advise against the use of "he/she" in scientific texts, we cannot do without it completely. However, it is undoubtedly good advice to use this and other slash combinations as sparingly as possible.

> ● *Gender neutral*: A study nurse will determine your blood pressure before and after the infusion. *He/she* will inform the study director of any abnormalities.

> ! Use the plural "they" if you refer to both women and men. If this is inappropriate, use "he/she" to include both sexes.

Another aspect of sexist writing concerns the use of marital titles. While men in our society have always been "Mr" (a title that does not reveal their marital status), women are labeled with respect to their marital status by using the term "Miss" for unmarried women and "Mrs" for married women.

I cannot think of any good reason why the neutral term "Ms," created in 1950 to include both unmarried and married women, should not be used. After years of resistance, most publishers and official bodies have meanwhile accepted this title.

> ! Use the neutral title (Ms) for women of either marital status, unless the woman holds a doctorate, in which case you should address her as "Dr."

Gender-biased expressions in scientific and medical literature are particularly annoying. How often do we still see the term "chairman" used for a woman chairing a scientific session? Similarly, a female speaker may be called a "spokesman," totally disregarding her gender. Such gender-marked terms are clearly unacceptable, and most of these can be easily replaced by a gender-neutral term.

When using general terms in connection with our fellow creatures, e.g., man, mankind, or manpower, a gender-neutral expression is always preferred. Here, this could be the human race, people, and workforce or staff.

> ! Use gender-neutral terms in titles and salutations. Avoid any expression containing "man" if you refer to both women and men.

8.3 Racist Writing

Race and ethnicity are cultural constructs, but they can have biological implications. Certain diseases occur exclusively or predominantly in a specific ethnic group, for example sickle cell anemia in persons with African ancestry or lactose intolerance in Chinese or Japanese subjects. Thus, it may be important to specify the race or ethnicity of subjects to whom a scientific or medical finding applies. Authors should explain and justify racial designators used, and such terms should be used accurately. This requires authors to be sensitive to the designations that individuals and groups prefer. Moreover, authors should be aware that designations may be handled differently by different organizations or journal editors, and that preferences may change over time.

> ! Use valid and politically correct racial or ethnic designations. Mention race and ethnicity only if this information is relevant to the scientific/medical message.

8.4 Ageism

Discrimination based on age is "ageism" and usually concerns older people. Bear in mind that "old" and "young" are relative terms. In the eyes of children, subjects beyond the age of 30 years tend to be "old," while a middle-aged person considers the 30-year olds as young. With increasing age, the division between young and old tends to shift.

In studies that involve humans, age should always be given specifically. Whenever possible, avoid general terms, such as "old people" or "the elderly." In studies involving a geriatric population, the term "geriatric" should be defined. Similarly, if findings apply to young subjects, "young" should be defined (e.g., subjects <20 years of age).

Sticking to Your Word: Avoiding Plagiarism

9

> *"If you steal from one author it's plagiarism;*
> *if you steal from many it's research."*
>
> Wilson Mizner

9.1 What Is Plagiarism?

When we drafted our first research manuscripts as young university students, our PhD supervisors' advice was, "Don't re-invent the wheel! Use the literature as published for all general parts of the paper."

In those days, no one paid much attention to the exact wording, provided the statements were appropriate and correct. A word-by-word statement taken from other researchers' publications did not upset anyone, as long as the statement ended with the reference to the original paper. In the meantime, however, the term "plagiarism" has become rather ubiquitous. The fear of a plagiarism accusation is palpable among my students, particularly since the recent scandals in connection with well-known public persons. Moreover, we have all become fully aware of the modern tools that will inevitably bring to light any attempt to present the work of others as our own.

But do we really understand what plagiarism means in the context of biomedical reporting? The *New Shorter Oxford English Dictionary* defines plagiarism as "the taking and using as one's own … the thoughts, writings, or inventions of another." In other words, plagiarism is implying that something is ours when it is not. It is the practice of claiming original authorship of texts or other creations, in their entirety or in part. This includes illustrations, ideas, images, and data.

In my experience, most scientists accused of plagiarism are completely unaware of their "crime." We may unwittingly imply, rather than claim, ownership of work or data, simply because we have failed to provide adequate acknowledgement of their source. Thus, plagiarism is concerned with false, insufficient, or missing attribution, in contrast to forgery in which the genuineness and authenticity of a document or other product are in question.

As you will appreciate, the section on plagiarism was one of the hardest for me to write. Almost every sentence on plagiarism I commit to paper may itself be plagiarism. I almost longed for the "good old days" when things were much easier, when the Internet did not exist and plagiarism was merely a Latin term occasionally encountered in connection with playwrights, songwriters, or poets who claimed that others had stolen their original work.

9.2 Forms of Plagiarism

Inevitably, the rapid and widespread dissemination of scientific findings via the Internet has provided an ideal breeding ground for plagiarism. The forms of plagiarism encountered are manifold, but the most common ones in scientific literature are plagiarism of text, plagiarism of ideas, and even self-plagiarism.

The nature of scientific communication is such that distinction between plagiarism of text and plagiarism of ideas is not always possible. Nonetheless, it makes sense to look at these two forms of scientific misconduct in closer detail.

9.2.1 Plagiarism of Text

The *AMA Manual of Style* considers four common forms of plagiarism of text, i.e., direct plagiarism, mosaic plagiarism, paraphrasing, and insufficient acknowledgement. They define direct plagiarism as the word-by-word transfer of text passages without the use of quotation marks or reference citations, while mosaic plagiarism is postulated to result if authors intertwine their ideas, words, and/or phrases with those of other authors without mentioning them. Paraphrasing is the restating of phrases or passages in a modified way without referring to the original author. According to the *AMA Manual of Style*, insufficient acknowledgement occurs if the source of only part of the borrowed text is disclosed, or if the description of the source material is insufficient for readers to distinguish between original and borrowed material.

Clearly, in literary work where the word itself is the artistic creation, e.g., in poetry, prose, journalism, plays, and songs, plagiarism of text is tantamount to blatant theft. In scientific publications, however, the originality lies in the scientific findings rather than the words used to describe them. For this reason, scientists tend to be overly careless and may use previously published text too liberally. Furthermore, many scientists report their research results in a language other than their native tongue, which poses an even greater challenge if plagiarism of text is to be avoided completely. This phenomenon is particularly noticeable in sections detailing the methods and procedures used. In an effort to save time and avoid mistakes, non-English speakers may be tempted to copy entire Methods sections from published work, frequently unaware that this is plagiarism of text.

In their rather nice Lancet article entitled "Rules of the game of scientific writing: fair play and plagiarism," Vessal and Habibzadeh (2007) call upon editors and reviewers to be more lenient towards authors of non-English origin, especially those in developing countries with limited access to professional editorial assistance. They urge readers and reviewers to make allowances for the occurrence of such "faux pas," as they call it, and suggest that the critics would probably not do a better job if called upon to write a scientific article in a foreign language.

> ! Place all specific terms or messages/conclusions taken from another author within quotation marks and acknowledge the exact source by giving the reference. Better: use your own words!

9.2.2 Plagiarism of Ideas

Plagiarism of ideas is the use of someone else's thought, hypothesis, conclusion, or interpretation in a way that implies it is entirely ours. Sometimes, plagiarism of ideas is masked by subtle or superficial modification of the original thought, with any reference to its author omitted.

Because scientific work in any discipline relies on ethical principles, the reporting of findings must equally be based on ethical thinking. This demands that any concept, result, or interpretation taken from other people's work must be properly acknowledged. In other words, our own contribution to the available literature should never be inflated with other researchers' findings, unless we make the source of the information absolutely clear.

The form for acknowledgment of other scientists' work varies between different journals and documents, but the typical approach is by using reference citations (see Sect. 7.2). In other types of text, e.g., legal documents, newspaper articles, or essays, footnotes are commonly used.

A scientific paper, however short, that provides no references to published literature is virtually unthinkable. The essence of scientific reporting is to place our own findings in the context of the existing knowledge created by others. While giving credit to our fellow scientists for their published findings is usually unproblematic, acknowledging other people's ideas is considerably trickier. Many of our brilliant ideas are born when we discuss our work with others, and retrospectively, it may be difficult to determine whether the idea was ours or someone else's. And how do you credit your 12-year old daughter for having a brilliant thought that leads to a completely new idea on your part?

Even the most ethical writers may occasionally fall in the trap of inadvertently using someone else's idea as their own. Such writers may be fully convinced that their idea was entirely their own, although the same notion or concept had previously been postulated by others. And where is the boundary between an original thought and the result of careful research? In the light of today's liberal exchange of scientific ideas, a truly original thought is almost nonexistent.

Although plagiarism of ideas tends to be unintentional, there are, unfortunately, cases of deliberate and malicious violation of scientific ethics. We all know of scientists, even Nobel Prize winners, who were given credit for discoveries that were in fact made by someone else. Moreover, the current system of peer-reviewed manuscripts adopted by many journals harbors considerable potential for plagiarism of ideas. Because selected referees (peers) tend to be involved in the same scientific area, they may derive important information and interesting new ideas from the unpublished work of others. Such referees should decline the review of manuscripts that are too closely related to their own research interests, on the grounds of a conflict of interest.

> ! Always acknowledge the contributions of others and the source of their ideas.

9.2.3 Self-Plagiarism

Scientists are under considerable pressure to publish as many papers as possible each year. Most of us know the rather apt saying, "publish or perish!" Moreover, the speed at which publications are being submitted and published is critical to the career advancement of scientists and their chances of research grant funding. Consequently, the temptation to indulge in self-plagiarism is understandable, at least in theory.

While we have a fairly clear picture of plagiarism of ideas or text, the concept of self-plagiarism is less well defined. Usually, self-plagiarism implies the renewed use of parts of our own publication in subsequent research papers. The most serious form of self-plagiarism is the resubmission of a previously published paper in which only the title and formatting have been altered. However, experienced scientists are aware of such misconduct and know that acts of self-plagiarism will not remain undetected.

The more common form of self-plagiarism consists of papers compiled from various sections of the author's own work already published. In some situations, this may be legitimate for certain parts of a publication, for example Methods sections that may, in fact, have remained unchanged in a subsequent study. However, if large parts of a paper are identical to previously published material, the credibility of both the paper and the author is in danger.

Many scientists argue that reusing their own texts is not objectionable because they do not "steal" from others. Such authors may make a good case for the necessity to "recycle" previous reports because they wish to reach a different audience or would like to place their scientific message in a somewhat altered context. The scientific community, however, does not share this notion. Arguments against self-plagiarism include unfairness, competition with more deserving publications, and unnecessary crowding of the literature with duplicated material. It is true to say that near-identical papers make it more difficult for others to find information relevant to a specific topic because much of it may simply be reiteration.

In a nice editorial published in 2009, editors of The Lancet ask the question, "Self-plagiarism: unintentional, harmless, or fraud?" The editors make a clear distinction between original research and review material when defining self-plagiarism. While they strongly censure the republishing of large parts of an original research paper as well as the use of isolated parts of the same study with near-identical Introduction and Methods sections in different journals, they argue that self-plagiarism in review or opinion papers is less harmful. Nonetheless, the editors claim that recycling existing text in review articles is still an attempt to deceive editors and readers. In this respect, it is unethical and constitutes intellectual laziness at best.

> ! Avoid self-plagiarism by refraining from recycling previously published material.

9.3 How to Avoid Plagiarism

All forms of plagiarism described above constitute an attempt to deceive the readers and thus amount to a serious form of scientific misconduct. You would agree that this should not be tolerated by the scientific community.

But how can we be sure that we do not fall victim to plagiarism, intentionally or unintentionally? Many high schools and universities have started to teach their students plagiarism prevention skills and how to safeguard themselves against accusations of plagiarism. Students are instructed to use a program that screens their texts for the presence of any plagiarized parts. Similarly, editors of many scientific journals routinely use programs to screen manuscripts submitted for publication. Examples of such programs are Turnitin designed by four UC Berkeley students (see http://turnitin.com) or CrossCheck powered by iThenticate (see www.ithenticate.com), but many other programs are available, several of them free of charge.

Publications involving multiple authors may be particularly at risk of containing plagiarized parts. Not every contributor may be aware of the implications of plagiarism, which can cause unexpected difficulties for the main author. Therefore, the main author is advised to screen the final manuscript for any plagiarized sections by using an appropriate program, e.g., DOC Cop (see www.doccop.com), prior to submission.

To protect yourself from accusations of plagiarism, make careful notes of the sources of all data and other materials used in your manuscript. Any specific term or message taken from another author must be placed within quotation marks, and the exact source must be acknowledged. Here is an example of quoted text:

> ● The authors concluded that "endoprosthetic treatment of proximal humeral fractures, both primary and secondary, leads to satisfactory results" [1].

However, quotation marks tend to be disruptive to the reader. Besides, it is often difficult to decide which portion of the original text to place between quotation marks because part of the statement may qualify for so-called shared language, i.e., words and phrases commonly used by the scientific community. It is thus advisable to use your own words to describe someone else's idea or outcome and add the appropriate reference.

Using your own words means, however, much more than paraphrasing the existing text. Let us look at an example:

> ● *Original text*: In our study, 26 of the 28 migraine patients reported a clear reduction of migraine attacks after 2 months of treatment with XYZ, and only one patient reported dizziness as an adverse event.
>
> *Paraphrased text*: In another study, 26 of the 28 migraine patients had considerably fewer migraine attacks after 2 months of treatment with XYZ. Moreover, only one patient experienced dizziness as an adverse event [1].

The second sentence is merely a semantic modification of the original sentence. Although the reference to the original source is given, the sentence was just paraphrased and would thus still be regarded as plagiarized.

Let us look at a version that would probably pass as "legitimately paraphrased":

> ● Miller et al. reported that 26 of 28 migraine patients benefited from a 2-month therapy with XYZ, with the frequency of migraine attacks clearly lower at the end of treatment [1]. In their study, XYZ was well tolerated, with dizziness experienced by a single patient [1].

Clearly, if you integrate information from your own study into previous findings from other studies, the risk of plagiarism is reduced:

> ● Our findings are in good agreement with those from previous studies in which XYZ was efficacious and well tolerated in patients suffering from migraine [1, 2, 3].

In summary, the best way to avoid plagiarism in scientific text is to fully understand the material under discussion. By "digesting" the information using our own way of thinking, the words used to describe other researchers' findings will become our own.

Structuring Scientific Texts: Getting the "Story" out

10

> "The secret of getting ahead is getting started. The secret of getting started is breaking your complex overwhelming tasks into small manageable tasks, and then starting on the first one."
>
> Mark Twain

10.1 Determining the Audience

When we write, we write for an assumed audience. This may be a community that is highly specialized in the area we are concerned with, or it may be a rather heterogeneous population of readers with varying levels of expertise in the field. By the style of writing we choose, we may intentionally or unintentionally include or exclude certain readers.

The effort of writing about our scientific findings only makes sense if the information reaches the intended audience. For this reason, we need to have a fairly clear concept of the targeted readers. How much knowledge on the subject can we assume? What level of detail is needed to place our "story" in the context of what is already known on the topic?

Many science writers are concerned that they may patronize, or even offend, their readers by providing excessive groundwork information. On the assumption that all learned readers know our topic as well as we do, we may skip important facts and findings that would have helped the readers to follow our train of thoughts. In my experience, most readers appreciate it to be guided along to some extent, even though the subject may not be new to them. Thus, the danger of boring the readers with facts they know already is minimal.

10.2 Adapting the "Story" to the Readers' Needs

Effective communication, i.e., communication that achieves the intended purpose, requires that we deliver our message in a way that can be grasped and understood by the targeted audience. Much of that concerns the structuring of scientific text. Many readers may specifically look for information concerning the methods used, or they may be particularly interested in the conclusions drawn from the study. By presenting the material in a logical and clear structure, we help our readers to readily find the information they need.

Thus, proper structuring of scientific manuscripts adds much value to their ease of "digestion." Remember that your paper or report has the highest chance of being read if its contents make sense to the reader, i.e., if the "story" is presented in a logical order. This implies that there is a clear beginning and clear ending, with an interesting, informative part in between.

The following techniques are helpful when drafting journal articles and other research reports:

- *Use a short and informative title*: If permitted by the chosen journal or other recipient of your manuscript, reveal conclusions in the title. For example, use a title such as "Treatment A is Superior to Treatment B in Children Suffering from Acute Leukemia," rather than "An Evaluation of Treatments A and B in Children Suffering from Acute Leukemia." Do, however, bear in mind that not all journal editors or organizers of scientific symposia encourage this type of title; it is therefore important to consult the relevant guidelines in advance. The running title should be a shortened version of the main title and should emphasize the main aspects of the study. The example above could be shortened to "Treatment of Acute Leukemia."
- *Prepare an interesting and self-contained abstract*: The abstract usually gets more attention than any other section of your article; in fact, it is often the only part readers are prepared to read. Therefore, the abstract should pique the readers' curiosity and encourage them to read the complete article. However, the abstract must never contain any information that is not detailed in the main part of the paper (see also Sect. 10.3).
- *Use IMRAD*: Give busy readers a chance to scan for information by organizing your text under headings such as Introduction, Methods and Materials, Results, and Discussion. This structure is commonly referred to as the IMRAD structure, with IMRAD used as an acronym made up from the first letters of the full terms plus an added "A" for "and." Some journals use modifications of the standard IMRAD, e.g., Objectives or Background for Introduction; Design, Setting, or Procedures for Methods and Materials; Outcome Measures or Findings for Results; and Conclusions for Discussion. Make sure you are familiar with the structure required by the journal you have in mind.
- *Pay utmost attention to the opening section* (*Introduction or Background*): State clearly what the article is about. Do not overwhelm readers with technical terms and jargons (see also Sect. 10.1). Avoid generalized or vague statements that could cover almost any topic. An opening sentence such as "This article is an

attempt to contribute to the ongoing debate in an important medical area" is of little interest to the reader.
- *Give a focused and accurate account of the methods used*: Provide enough information on all materials and methods used, including statistical tests and other analyses, to enable an interested reader to reproduce the experiment or study and to verify the reported results. Do not report any results in the Methods section.
- *Clearly separate the results from the discussion*: Describe your findings in the Results section and save their interpretation for the discussion. Actual numbers (e.g., rates, percentages, *P* values) stated in the Results section should not be restated in the Discussion section. In general, the Discussion section should address the findings in a qualitative sense, but it may occasionally be necessary to highlight individual values to make the intended point. The Discussion section should primarily focus on interpreting the findings in the context of the existing knowledge. Moreover, the implication of newly gained knowledge and consequences for future research should be addressed in the Discussion section.
- *Keep the conclusions short and focused*: Present the conclusions in a clear, concise language so that your results are easily understood. Do not draw any conclusions that go beyond the reported data. Extensive hypothesizing merely emphasizes the lack of clear conclusions and shows up uncertainty on the part of the author.

10.3 Drafting an Abstract

10.3.1 The Importance of Abstracts

In recent years, access to scientific data has become very easy, and abstracts tend to be freely available. Because abstracts are important to direct readers to articles of interest, the abstract should be enticing and compelling. This requires that the abstract be written in a clear and simple language using the appropriate tense (mostly past tense for work done). If the abstract is confusing or vague, the readers will probably not go on reading the full paper. In addition, most journals limit the number of words in the abstract to 250 or 300, which necessitates a brief and concise writing style.

An abstract should be viewed as a mini version of the paper (or scientific poster), summarizing the main points of each section. Moreover, it should be a self-contained summary of the study and should never give information or conclusions not supported by the data shown. In addition, references to literature should be avoided except in rare instances, e.g., if a modified version of a previously published method was used and reference to the original method is of interest.

Generally, an abstract should not contain any abbreviations or acronyms, unless they are more commonly known than the full term or if the term is mentioned several times in the abstract. In this case, define the term on first mention and thereafter use the abbreviation.

Typically, we use two types of abstracts, i.e., the descriptive abstract and informative abstract. These are described below.

10.3.2 Descriptive Abstracts

Descriptive abstracts tend to be short (≤ 100 words) and solely indicate the type of information found in the paper. They do not provide any results, conclusions, or recommendations. A descriptive abstract does not evaluate or judge the results of the study. It may be considered an outline of the work or a table of contents presented in sentences.

A descriptive abstract merely summarizes the purpose and scope of the study and usually states the methods used to arrive at the reported findings. While readers do not learn anything about the outcome of the study, they are informed about the contents of the paper.

10.3.3 Informative Abstracts

Informative abstracts are the more common type of abstracts used. They are longer than descriptive abstracts; most journals allow 250 words, with some limiting the word count to 150 words or 300 words. Depending on the journal, the informative abstract can be a single paragraph without structuring or may be structured using the IMRAD layout (see also Sect. 10.3.4).

In addition to the information given in a descriptive abstract, the informative abstract summarizes the results and conclusions of the study. If well prepared, this type of abstract is a mini version of the full paper, with the most important aspects of the study summarized.

10.3.4 Structured Abstracts

Several studies have shown that structured abstracts are more effective than unstructured abstracts. This means that such abstracts are more frequently consulted than unstructured ones, and their contents are more readily understood. The headings used in a structured abstract are essentially those used in the main part of the manuscript. Thus, use IMRAD or an adapted structure, in line with the instructions for authors of the journal you have in mind.

Some journals do not explicitly request a structured abstract. Nevertheless, it may be helpful to structure your abstract even for such journals because it is considerably easier to write if clear headings are in place. The journal editors may subsequently change the format at their discretion.

Appendix

11.1 Scientific Writing Rules at a Glance

TOPIC	RULES
Scientific communication	Successful communication in science involves clarity and simplicity, short sentences, transparency, and consistency.
	Biomedical communicators and scientific writers do not need to "dumb down" scientific writing or omit technical terms to write plainly and clearly. However, they do need to define or explain terms that their audiences may not recognize. They also need to write logically, building from what information the reader knows to what new information the reader will learn in the article.
	Quantity can never replace quality of our scientific message, nor can it mask any vagueness we may have because of an incomplete understanding of the concepts.
Spelling	Misspelled words in sciences distract and annoy the reader. The credibility of your work hinges on the proper use of the language.
	Every document that leaves the writer's desk must have undergone careful screening for spelling errors, both by the author/editor and the spell checker.
	A mixture of American and British spelling within any one document is both confusing and annoying to the reader.
	If you have the choice, use either American or British spelling, but do so consistently. Keep your target audience in mind (European versus international).
	If language requirements are defined (e.g., company-internal conventions, journal house style, publishers' requirements), use the given spelling rules consistently.

(continued)

TOPIC	RULES
Punctuation	*Do not hyphenate Latin expressions or non–English-language phrases used in an adjectival sense, e.g.,* in vivo *experiments,* a priori *argument.*
	In the text, do not use hyphens to express a range (e.g., 10% to 20% of the substance), except if the range expresses fiscal years or life spans (e.g., the 1975–1982 data set) or if the range is given in parentheses (e.g., mean age was 22 years; [range, 11–32 years]).
	Do not hyphenate modifiers in which the second element is a number or letter, e.g., type 2 diabetes, grade A material.
	Divide words only if necessary, and divide them correctly.
	Never use contractions in medical, scientific, technical, or other professional texts.
	Use nonbreaking spaces and hyphens to avoid inappropriate separation of terms.
Shortened word forms	*Define abbreviations the first time they appear. Subsequently, use the abbreviation rather than the full term.*
	Avoid abbreviations in titles and abstracts, as well as at the beginning of a sentence (unless the full term is cumbersome or excessively lengthy).
	Use a glossary of abbreviations (unless this is not encouraged by the journal to which you wish to submit your paper).
	Use units of measurement consistently (e.g., ml or mL). Use the same abbreviations for the singular and plural forms (e.g., 1 mL, 10 mL; 1 h, 3 h; 1 cm, 50 cm).
	Use capitals and no periods (full stops) for acronyms and initialisms. Exceptions are words that have become commonly accepted as nouns (e.g., laser, scuba).
	Do not capitalize the words from which an acronym or initialism is derived (e.g., prostate-specific antigen [PSA]).
	Use no apostrophe in plural forms (e.g., ECGs, RBCs).
	Suspensions (e.g., Mr, Dr) do not have to be followed by a period. True abbreviations (e.g., Prof.), however, always end with a period.
Numbers	*Getting your numbers right first time saves much time and effort in subsequent editing rounds.*
	Spell out one-digit numbers (one to nine), and use numerals for all larger numbers.
	Whatever style of expressing numbers you adopt, remember to be consistent. Heterogeneous styles in any single document are both distracting and annoying to the reader.
Capitalization	*Capitalized words in science are either proper nouns, key words in titles, or first words of sentences.*
Tense	*Report established knowledge in the present tense but new, previously unpublished findings (including your own results) in the past tense.*

(continued)

11.1 Scientific Writing Rules at a Glance

TOPIC	RULES
Parallel statements	*For parallelism, the terms linked via a conjunction must have the same grammatical structure.*
Subject–verb agreement	*In general, a singular subject takes a singular verb, and a plural subject takes a plural verb.*
	For terms that can be either singular or plural, use the singular verb if the term refers to a unit, amount, discipline, or organization. Use the plural verb if the term indicates individual members or components rather than the collection as a whole.
Syntax (word order)	*Modifying phrases should be as close as possible to the words, phrases, or clauses they modify.*
	If the adverb strongly qualifies the verb, i.e., if you wish to place special emphasis on the nature of the action, it is legitimate to split the infinitive.
	Although you may end a sentence with a preposition, place the preposition within the sentence if the same meaning is achieved.
Danglers	*Carefully check proper participle–subject matching in sentences that include a participle.*
	Avoid dangling gerunds by using an alternative noun and proper word order.
Respectively	*Only use "respectively" if two series are listed and if there could be ambiguity. Use a comma before "respectively".*
Plurals of abstractions and attributes	*Use the singular for abstractions and attributes possessed in common.*
Active voice	*Use the active voice most of the time because it is more direct and less wordy. If you want to emphasize the action rather than the agent, use the passive voice, bearing in mind that the proportion of passive verbs should not exceed 30%.*
Copula formulations	*Copula formulations are frequently essential. However, a powerful alternative for the verb "to be" may sometimes make the sentence more interesting.*
Prepositions	*Use prepositions in a "healthy" proportion to the remaining words of the sentence (i.e., no more than one preposition per four words).*
Modifiers	*Use modifiers in moderation. Limit the number of decorative words to those that add necessary information to the statement.*
	Avoid modifier strings in sentences, names, and titles.
Uniform Requirements and journal house style	*Before drafting a manuscript, consult the current version of the Uniform Requirements as well as the specific instructions for authors of the selected journal.*
Company-internal conventions	*Poor writing style handed down by tradition will delay review of the document. This, in turn, prolongs the "time to market" of publications and applications for marketing authorization of new drugs. An internal style manual to be used by all contributors can be a great help.*
Double negatives	*If the statement is positive, state it in the positive.*
Tautology	*Do not duplicate terms and expressions.*
Jargonized writing	*Resist the temptation to use jargon in scientific writing. Always apply your common sense before adopting a term from others.*

(continued)

TOPIC	RULES
Oxymorons	When using an oxymoron, make sure the term is commonly known and its use is appropriate in scientific communication.
Reference style	When quoting published or unpublished information, consult the journal's house style and follow the reference style consistently. If no specific guidelines are given, use Vancouver style.
Sexist writing	Use the plural "they" if you refer to both women and men. If this is inappropriate, use "he/she" to include both sexes. Use the neutral title (Ms) for women of either marital status, unless the woman holds a doctorate, in which case you should address her as "Dr." Use gender-neutral terms in titles and salutations. Avoid any expression containing "man" if you refer to both women and men.
Racist writing	Use valid and politically correct racial or ethnic designations. Mention race and ethnicity only if this information is relevant to the scientific/medical message.
Plagiarism	Always acknowledge the contributions of others and the source of their ideas. Place all specific terms or messages/conclusions taken from another author within quotation marks and acknowledge the exact source by giving the reference. Better: use your own words! Avoid self-plagiarism by refraining from recycling previously published material.

11.2 American English Versus British English: Groups of Words Affected by the Different Spelling

DIFFERENCES	AMERICAN	BRITISH
or for our	color endeavor humor tumor	colour endeavour humour tumour
e for oe	celiac diarrhea edema esophagus estrogen fetus	coeliac diarrhoea oedema oesophagus oestrogen foetus
e for ae	anemia anesthetic cecum etiology hematuria hemoglobin pediatric	anaemia anaesthetic caecum aetiology haematuria haemoglobin paediatric

(continued)

DIFFERENCES	AMERICAN	BRITISH
–er for –re	center	centre
	meter	metre
	theater	theatre
–ize for –ise	analyze	analyse
	catheterize	catheterise
	criticize	criticise
	sensitize	sensitise
–ization for –isation	organization	organisation
	liberalization	liberalisation
–al omitted	anatomic	anatomical
	histologic	histological
	physiologic	physiological
	logic	logical
f for ph	sulfonamide	sulphonamide
	sulfur	sulphur
single l for double l	beveled	bevelled
	traveled	travelled
	labeled	labelled
single s for double s	focused	focussed
single t for double t	targeted	targetted
silent endings omitted	catalog	catalogue
	gram	gramme
	program	programme

11.3 The Main Punctuation Marks in Scientific Writing

PUNCTUATION MARK	SYMBOL	…AND HOW TO USE IT PROPERLY
Comma	,	*After an introductory word (often an adverb) in a sentence*: – Subsequently, we stained the immunoblots. – However, the difference was not statistically significant. *To set off a nonessential clause*: – Scientists, who often work overtime, tend to lack the time for writing manuscripts. *After an introductory (prepositional or adverbial) phrase*: – Generally speaking, this is sound advice. *To separate two independent clauses in a compound sentence*: – All blood samples were processed, and IgG levels were determined. *To set off appositives or interrupting words*: – Alzheimer's disease, named after Dr. Alois Alzheimer, is the most common form of dementia.

(continued)

PUNCTUATION MARK	SYMBOL	...AND HOW TO USE IT PROPERLY
Serial comma (also called Oxford comma)	,	Before "*and*" or "*or*" in a series of at least three items: – The nature, intensity, and relationship to trial medication of each adverse event were reported. – Any patient willing to continue with treatment, showing tumor regression, or exhibiting disease stabilization was included in the study.
Hyphen	-	*To link two words jointly modifying a third*: – a pale-yellow granular substance; a single-center, double-blind clinical study; low-quality raw material NOTE: *Do not hyphenate word combinations involving adverbs.* – freshly collected samples, fully informed patients, markedly reduced production cost *To avoid confusion*: – The dentist's chair was re-covered. *In spelled-out compound numbers*: – twenty-one to fifty-five times *With number modifiers*: – a 20-year old subject, a 2-year study *In words containing a prefix or suffix*: – anti-inflammatory, pre-existing, a follow-up study NOTE: *Hyphens are no longer necessary for prefixes such as intra, inter, pre, post, non, re, or sub, except if two vowels meet.* –intrasubject variation, nonessential clause, postdosing events, recalculated data
Semicolon	;	*To link two independent clauses if a sense of "anticipation" is appropriate*: – There are a number of test kits available; however, the standard products are used in most cases. NOTE: *Semicolons should be used sparingly. If possible, use comma or period (full stop) instead of semicolon.*
Colon	:	*Use only if a sentence or paragraph introduces the text that follows*: – The methods used were as follows: ... NOTE: *Do not use colons within sentences.*
Apostrophe	'	*To show possession*: – the chemist's bench, Newton's law, the pharmacists' reunion NOTE: *To a plural not ending in "s," add an apostrophe and an "s."* – the children's parents *With units of time or money if applied as possessive adjectives*: – of two days' duration, in a few hours' time, 10 cents' worth of advice, 20 years' clinical experience
Slash (virgule)	/	*To indicate "and," "or," or "per"*: – he/she, and/or, 20 mg/L NOTE: *Avoid constructions such as 20 mg/L of NaCl. Reword: NaCl concentration of 20 mg/L.*

(continued)

11.4 Awkward Phrases to Avoid

PUNCTUATION MARK	SYMBOL	...AND HOW TO USE IT PROPERLY
Quotation marks	"..."	*To highlight a term*: – The term "pyrexia" replaces the word "fever" throughout the report. *NOTE: In English, both quotation marks are placed above the word.* *To enclose a direct quotation*: – The physician asked, "How are you feeling today?" *NOTE: If you quote material exceeding four typewritten lines, set it off in a block using reduced type size and omit the quotation marks.*
Punctuation and quotation marks	"..."	*Place periods and commas inside quotation marks*: – All students had read "Faust." – Use the "Instructions for Authors," as they tend to give good advice. *Place semicolons and colons outside closing quotation marks*: – Below is a definition of the population termed "evaluable for efficacy": *Place question marks or exclamation points inside quotation marks only when the quotation itself is a direct question or an exclamation. Otherwise, place these marks outside*: – The physician asked at regular intervals, "How have you been since the last visit?"
Single quotation marks	'...'	*Use single quotation marks for quotations within quotations*: – She looked at her students and said, "As my teacher always pointed out, 'Scientific writing can be fun,' and I agree."
Ellipses (*three spaced dots*)	. . .	*To indicate omission of one or more words, lines, paragraphs, or data from quoted material*: – The results indicated ... good agreement between the two methods used. *At the end of a sentence, ellipses follow the final punctuation mark (the final punctuation mark is set close to the preceding word.)*: – All differences tested were statistically significant....

11.4 Awkward Phrases to Avoid

AWKWARD PHRASES	PREFERRED EXPRESSIONS
a majority of	*most*
a number of	*many*
a sufficient amount of	*enough*
according to our data	*we find / we found*
accordingly	*therefore, so*
after the conclusion of / after termination of	*after*
along the lines of	*like, such as*

(continued)

AWKWARD PHRASES	PREFERRED EXPRESSIONS
are of the same opinion	*agree*
as is the case	*as is true*
ascertain the location of	*find*
at such time as	*when*
at that point in time	*then*
at the present time	*now*
at this point in time	*now*
based on the fact that	*because*
be deficient in	*lack*
be in a position to	*can, be able*
by a factor of two	*double, twice*
by means of	*by*
come to a conclusion	*conclude*
despite the fact that	*although*
due to the fact that	*because*
during the time that	*while*
equally as well	*as well, equally well*
fewer in number	*fewer*
first of all	*first*
for the purpose of	*to, for*
for the reason that	*because*
for this reason	*thus, therefore*
give consideration to	*consider, examine*
give indication of	*show, indicate, suggest*
happen(s) to be	*is / are*
has been proved to be	*is*
has the capability of	*can*
if conditions are such that	*if*
in a number of	*several, many*
in all cases	*always*
in case	*if*
in close proximity to	*near*
in excess of	*more than*
in large measure	*largely*
in many cases	*often*
in most cases	*usually*
in my opinion	*I think*
in no case	*never*
in order that	*so that*
in order to	*to*
in some cases	*sometimes*
in terms of	*in*
in the amount of	*for*
in the case of	*for*

(continued)

11.4 Awkward Phrases to Avoid

AWKWARD PHRASES	PREFERRED EXPRESSIONS
in the event that	if
in the field of	in
in the near future	soon
in the neighborhood of	near, about, nearly, approx.
in the order of	about, approximately
in the vicinity of	near
in this case	here
in view of the fact that	because, since
is capable of	can
is found to be	is
is in a position to	can
it has been found that	it is
it has long been known that	it is
it is a fact that	it is
it is evident that	it is
it is interesting to note that	note that
it is noted that	it is
it is our opinion that	we think
it is possible that	perhaps
it is well known that	it is
it is worth pointing out	note that
it may, however, be noted that	but
lacked the ability to	could not, was not
make inquiry regarding	ask about, inquire about
manner in which	how
notwithstanding the fact that	although
on a daily basis	daily
on the basis of	from, because, by
perform	do
present in greater abundance	more abundant
provided that	if
put an end to	end
reach a conclusion	conclude
serves the function of being	is
subsequent to	after
take into consideration	consider
the question as to whether	whether
there can be little doubt that	probably
through the use of	by
utilize	use
utilization	use
with a view to	to
with reference to	about
with the exception	except

11.5 List of Academic Degrees and Honors

Note: The spelling of the degrees reflects the original British or American usage.

SHORT FORM	FULL TITLE
ART	Accredited record technician
Bs, BCh, BC, CB, or ChB	Bachelor of surgery
BSN	Bachelor of science in nursing
CNM	Certified nurse midwife
CNMT	Certified nuclear medicine technologist
CO	Certified orthoptist
COMT	Certified ophthalmic medical technologist
CPFT	Certified pulmonary function technologist
CRNA	Certified registered nurse anesthetist
CRTT	Certified respiratory therapy technician
DC	Doctor of chiropractic
DCh or ChD	Doctor of surgery
DDS	Doctor of dental surgery
DMD	Doctor of dental medicine
DME	Doctor of medical education
DMSc	Doctor of medical science
DNE	Doctor of nursing education
DNS or DNSc	Doctor of nursing science
DO or OD	Doctor of optometry
DO	Doctor of osteopathy
DPH or DrPH	Doctor of public health; doctor of public hygiene
DPharm	Doctor of pharmacy
DSW	Doctor of social work
DTM&H	Diploma in tropical medicine and hygiene
DTPH	Diploma in tropical pediatric hygiene
DVM, DMV, or VMD	Doctor of veterinary medicine
DVMS	Doctor of veterinary medicine and surgery
DVS or DVSc	Doctor of veterinary science
EdD	Doctor of education
ELS	Editor in the life sciences
EMT	Emergency medical technician
EMT-P	Emergency medical technician-paramedic
FCGP	Fellow of the College of General Practitioners
FCPS	Fellow of the College of Physicians and Surgeons
FFA	Fellow of the Faculty of Anaesthetists
FFARCS	Fellow of the Faculty of Anaesthetists of the Royal College of Surgeons
FNP	Family nurse practitioner
FP	Family practitioner
FRACP	Fellow of the Royal Australian College of Physicians
FRCGP	Fellow of the Royal College of General Practitioners
FRCOG	Fellow of the Royal College of Obstetricians and Gynaecologists
FRCP	Fellow of the Royal College of Physicians

(continued)

11.5 List of Academic Degrees and Honors

SHORT FORM	FULL TITLE
FRCPath	*Fellow of the Royal College of Pathologists*
FRCPC	*Fellow of the Royal College of Physicians of Canada*
FRCPE or FRCP(Edin)	*Fellow of the Royal College of Physicians of Edinburgh*
FRCP(Glasg)	*Fellow of the Royal College of Physicians and Surgeons of Glasgow qua Physician*
FRCPI or FRCP(Ire)	*Fellow of the Royal College of Physicians of Ireland*
FRCR	*Fellow of the Royal College of Radiologists*
FRCS	*Fellow of the Royal College of Surgeons*
FRCSC	*Fellow of the Royal College of Surgeons of Canada*
FRCSE or FRCS(Edin)	*Fellow of the Royal College of Surgeons of Edinburgh*
FRCS(Glasg)	*Fellow of the Royal College of Physicians and Surgeons of Glasgow qua Surgeon*
FRCSI or FRCS(Ire)	*Fellow of the Royal College of Surgeons of Ireland*
FRCVS	*Fellow of the Royal College of Veterinary Surgeons*
FRS	*Fellow of the Royal Society*
GNP	*Gerontologic or geriatric nurse practitioner*
JD	*Doctor of jurisprudence*
LLB	*Bachelor of laws*
LLD	*Doctor of laws*
LLM	*Master of laws*
LPN	*Licensed practical nurse*
LVN	*Licensed visiting nurse; licensed vocational nurse*
MA or AM	*Master of arts*
M(ASCP)	*Registered technologist in microbiology (American Society of Clinical Pathologists)*
MB or BM	*Bachelor of medicine*
MBA	*Master of business administration*
MBBS or MB,BS	*Bachelor of medicine, bachelor of surgery*
MD or DM	*Doctor of medicine*
ME	*Medical examiner*
MEd	*Master of education*
MHA	*Master of hospital administration*
MN	*Master of nursing*
MPA	*Master of public administration*
MPH	*Master of public health*
MPharm	*Master of pharmacy*
MRCP	*Member of the Royal College of Physicians*
MRCS	*Member of the Royal College of Surgeons*
MS, MSc, or SM	*Master of science*
MS, SM, MCh, MSurg	*Master of surgery*
MSN	*Master of science in nursing*
MSPH	*Master of science in public health*
MSW	*Master of social welfare; master of social work*
MT	*Medical technologist*
MTA	*Medical technical assistant*
MT(ASCP)	*Registered medical technologist (American Society of Clinical Pathologists)*
NP	*Nurse practitioner*

(continued)

SHORT FORM	FULL TITLE
OT	*Occupational therapist*
OTR	*Occupational therapist, registered*
PA	*Physician assistant*
PA-C	*Physician assistant, certified*
PharmD, DP, or PD	*Doctor of pharmacy*
PharmG	*Graduate in pharmacy*
PhD or Dphil	*Doctor of philosophy*
PNP	*Pediatric nurse practitioner*
PsyD	*Doctor of psychology*
PT	*Physical therapist*
RD	*Registered dietitian*
RN	*Registered nurse*
RNA	*Registered nurse anesthetist*
RNC or RN,C	*Registered nurse, certified*
RPFT	*Registered pulmonary function technologist*
RPh	*Registered pharmacist*
RPT	*Registered physical therapist*
RRL	*Registered record librarian*
RT	*Radiologic technologist; respiratory therapist*
RTR	*Recreational therapist, registered*
ScD, DSc, or DS	*Doctor of science*

From AMA Manual of Style: A Guide for Authors and Editors. 10th ed. Oxford University Press; 2009.

Exercises

12.1 Exercise 1 | Consistent Spelling

Correct any spelling errors in the following sentences, bearing the target audience in mind. Please note that some sentences need no correction.

SENTENCES CONTAINING SPELLING ERRORS
British journal: Clinical chemistry tests (i.e., hematocrit, haemoglobin, and hematuria) were performed at a single study center to minimize variability between laboratories.
American research report: All histological and histopathologic findings from the foetuses confirmed the presence of multiple oedemas.
European clinical study: This was a single-center, placebo-controlled study to determine the effects of the LH-RH analog on estrogen levels in a pediatric population with central precocious puberty.
International textbook: The human brain is made up of billions of neurons. Each has a cell body, an axon, and many dendrites. The cell body contains a nucleus, which controls all of the cell's activities, and several other structures that perform specific functions. The axon, which is much, much narrower than the width of a human hair, extends out from the cell body and transmits messages to other neurons.

12.2 Exercise 2 | Proper Punctuation

Correct any punctuation errors in the following sentences. Please note that some sentences need no correction.

SENTENCES CONTAINING PUNCTUATION ERRORS
1. Moreover our findings are in good agreement, with published data
2. Medicinal materials, which are produced from bovine sources, are now being replaced by nonbovine materials.

(continued)

SENTENCES CONTAINING PUNCTUATION ERRORS
3. In general, scientific writing is an interesting task.
4. The committee members concluded, that the project is well-structured and should go ahead as planned.
5. The trial participants were below 20-years of age, and able to read, and understand the instructions.
6. We used a high precision-immunoassay.
7. All patients were followed-up after the end of treatment.
8. The markedly-improved manufacturing process resulted in a higher yield.
9. The company promises a 5 years shelf-life for the capsules.
10. This was a 5 months' study, with the follow up-phase lasting 2 months.
11. Both, a pro- and retrospective analysis were performed.
12. Although we have a competent staff; bottlenecks do occur.
13. The techniques used included: TLC, HPLC, and NMR.
14. "Nausea" was defined here as feeling "queasy" for longer than two hours.
15. Is that book your's?
16. The new antihypertensive drug represents a genuine advance owing to it's favorable pharmacokinetic profile.
17. The authors confirm that the data have not been published elsewhere [see author's signatures].
18. The concentration of stabilizer in the medium was 0.5 mg/L^{-1}.
19. The general practitioner is advised to refer his/her patients to an endocrinologist in such cases.
20. In our study, we used the novel imaging technique for the first time!
21. A deficiency of the trial was the limited number of plasma samples available for analysis — in fact, as many as 42% of samples were lost.
22. Scientific writers of a non-English-origin may have to consult a good dictionary at times.
23. The in-vitro findings agreed very well with the in-vivo results.
24. The incidence of metabolic syndrome in the USA is estimated to be as high as 30–40%.
25. Delayed growth was common in this pediatric population (with growth-hormone (GH) deficiency being the most frequent cause; in line with published literature (12, 13)).
26. Dr. P. Smith and Mr. A. Black were in charge.
27. The main authors were S. Green (Ph.D.) and T. Matthews (M.D.).
28. Our findings didn't reveal any connection between the increased heart rate and duration of drug intake.

12.3 Exercise 3 | Using Numbers and Percentages Correctly

Using the rules for writing numbers and expressing percentages, correct the following sentences:

SENTENCES CONTAINING ERRONEOUS NUMBERS
15 patients were enrolled in the clinical study in Spain.
A mean half-life of 2.5 h was calculated from the plasma concentrations of eight male and fourteen female rats.

(continued)

After a further 4 h, we added H₂O (five mL) and NADH (ten mL) to the incubation mixture.
The production campaign comprised lots of five, ten, and twenty kg of raw material.
The patient was released from hospital after 5 months.
After the left thoracotomy, dogs were allowed to recover for three days.
Of the seventy-one patients taking part in this survey, only twenty attended all study visits. 35 patients were lost to follow-up, and fifteen patients withdrew prematurely from the study. One patient died.
11% of the cells had to be discarded.
Intra-assay precision ranged from 89–99%.

12.4 Exercise 4 | Using Proper Capitalization

Using the rules for capitalizing words, correct the following sentences:

SENTENCES CONTAINING CAPITALIZATION ERRORS
Table heading: Patient data of Efficacy and tolerability – a summary
Study title: Follow-Up study of X-Ray findings in Patients who had Undergone brain Surgery
Serious adverse events occurring in more than 10% of patients are listed in table 2.
The new drug was tested in wistar rats, Cynomolgus monkeys, and Beagle Dogs.
The boy had Asperger Autism in addition to his Attention-deficit disorder.
In our study, Group A was clearly more responsive than Group B.
Genetic analysis revealed an impairment of Chromosome 21.
Method 1 proved more reliable than Method 2.

12.5 Exercise 5 | Using Tenses in Scientific Reporting

Consider the following sentences and label them "correct / incorrect" with respect to tense. Rewrite the sentences you consider incorrect.

SECTIONS AND SENTENCES	CORRECT	INCORRECT
Introduction: Similar findings were reported by Jones et al.		
Introduction: It has long been known that smoking increased the risk of cardiovascular disease.		
Methods: The method used for analysis of plasma concentrations of parent compound and metabolites is an HPLC technique with UV detection.		
Results: The epidemiological data collected in this clinical trial were listed in Table 1 of this report.		
Results: The subclones containing the D-helix substitutions were reassembled into plasmid P.		

(continued)

SECTIONS AND SENTENCES	CORRECT	INCORRECT
Discussion: In our study we find that there are significantly fewer CNS effects in mice receiving vehicle only than in those receiving the test compound.		
Discussion: Recently published work by Miller et al. [1] characterizes the chemical structure of this compound.		

12.6 Exercise 6 | Restoring Parallelism

Consider the following sentences and label them "correct / incorrect" with respect to parallelism. Correct the sentences you consider nonparallel.

NONPARALLEL SENTENCES	CORRECT	INCORRECT
Thus, for the study of effects on the composition of and/or mediated by colonic lipids, the rat apparently is an acceptable animal model.		
Under no circumstances was any subject enrolled for this study and completed the three treatments allowed to be randomized and enrolled for a second course of treatment.		
The book, written for chemists and laboratory technicians, is expected to be most useful.		
In the subgroup analysis, there were no relevant differences in the frequency of adverse events with regard to sex and in comparison with the whole population.		
Patients with stable disease or showing a complete or partial response, or if no disease progression is documented, may continue with the treatment until the planned study end.		
The American research group reported incidences that were superior and less variable than those reported elsewhere.		
The participating cardiologists reported that more than half of the diabetic patients suffering from hypertension were as easy to work with, required no more time to treat, and showed as good or better improvement than other hypertensive patients.		
When applying proper writing rules, you will save time, energy and feel satisfied with your work.		
The statistical method is described in 4.2 and the results reported in 5.2.		

12.7 Exercise 7 | Avoiding Verbal Phrase Danglers

Consider the following examples of danglers and correct the sentences by restoring the syntax (word order):

VERBAL PHRASE DANGLERS
Being the first member of the pharmacological class, the database of this ACE inhibitor served as a model.
Lying on top of the gut, you can see a thin tissue.
While having lunch, the reaction mixture exploded.
In analyzing the data statistically, the *Salmonella* infections were indeed rare.
Considering the observed pharmacodynamic effect, the data indicate a large safety margin for the active drug.
After introducing it in 1968, broad clinical application of trospium chloride in patients with either gastrointestinal disorders or urinary dysfunction proved it to be safe and efficacious.

12.8 Exercise 8 | Using "Respectively" Properly

Consider the sentences below and identify those where the use of "respectively" is unnecessary or even wrong:

SENTENCES CONTAINING "RESPECTIVELY"
Blood and urine samples were taken after 2 h and 4 h, respectively.
At Visit 1, subjects received the necessary drug supply, a micturition diary to be filled in twice a day, and a full study description to be signed at the next visit, respectively.
Validation data showed good agreement if generated in-house or by the external laboratory, respectively.
The bulk supply and quantities needed for the Phase III studies were both produced by Product GmbH, respectively.
The three referees commented on the poor quality of the figures, the confusing layout of some of the tables, and the incomplete description of the assay methods, respectively.
Values for t_{max} in rats, rabbits, and humans were 0.5 h, 1.4 h, and 3.8 h, respectively.

12.9 Exercise 9 | Avoiding Excessive Passive Voice

Consider the voice of the following sentences and mark them with an A for "active" or a P for "passive." Which ones of the passive sentences would be more powerful in the active voice? Recast the selected sentences in the active voice and comment on the change.

ACTIVE/PASSIVE SENTENCES	VOICE A/P
Treatment with a single tablet has been shown to be as effective as a 7-day therapy with the cream [1].	
Usually, centrifugation for 15 min suffices to separate the two layers.	
Immediately after the accident, the 80-year old woman was taken to the emergency department of the nearby hospital.	
According to Miller et al. [2], direct DNA binding of the compound is considered the most likely mechanism of mutagenic action.	
The opinion held by Hunter et al. is not shared by this author.	
After noninvasive tests, the final diagnosis of a breast tumor is made by biopsy.	
Subsequent magnetic resonance imaging supported our hypothesis.	
Test tubes used in clinical chemistry testing are made of glass.	
The behavior of the rats was monitored for 24 h by two independent technicians.	
None of the comparators used was shown to be more potent in this experimental system.	
Our findings are compared with literature data in Table 3.	
Statistical analysis did not indicate any significant difference between the two treatments.	

12.10 Exercise 10 | Limiting the Number of Prepositions

In the sentences below, identify the prepositions and determine the ratio of prepositions to other words. Recast the sentences to achieve a more acceptable ratio of prepositions to other words.

SENTENCES CONTAINING TOO MANY PREPOSITIONS
The information on qualitative method comparison of assays for drugs of abuse is summarized in the flowchart below.
The incidence of events of appetite suppression in children treated with Ritalin in a population of school children in the USA and in Canada is indicated in the table below.
The data from mutation assays were further analyzed in order to get to know more about the underlying mechanism.

12.11 Exercise 11 | Using Modifiers in Moderation

In the sentences below, identify the modifiers and classify them as adjectives, adverbs, or noun modifiers. Rewrite the sentences by retaining the essential modifiers and removing all "decorative" words.

SENTENCES CONTAINING TOO MANY MODIFIERS
Future proposed and essential changes to the currently applied validation process and for the ideal and suitable equipment will be thoroughly and extensively reviewed by the responsible process change committee.
This statistically significantly different result was more than surprising after the many convincing reports clearly documenting the absence of a marked drug effect.
We cannot fully and unambiguously explain the potentially underlying mechanism in the absence of more detailed technical analyses of this very interesting phenomenon.

12.12 Exercise 12 | Avoiding Tautological and Other Redundant Expressions

In the sentences below, identify the tautological and otherwise redundant expressions. Recast the sentences by removing any unnecessary words.

SENTENCES CONTAINING TAUTOLOGICAL OR REDUNDANT EXPRESSIONS
If a serious adverse event occurred, the study was immediately terminated prematurely.
The mice in the first experiment were heavier in weight than those in the second experiment.
For easy comparison, the results are plotted graphically.
The staining was red in color.
The finding may potentially indicate a possible relationship between product stability and enzyme activity.
Further work is needed to establish the true facts.
In none of the experiments was no immune reaction at all.
We were astonished by the end result.
The patient has no past history of suicides.
We believe that the potential hazards of this X-ray examination are extremely minimal.
The team reached a consensus of opinion before finalizing the protocol.
We selected the most unique clinical center for the study.

Solutions to Exercises

13.1 Solutions to Exercise 1

CORRECTED SENTENCES	COMMENTS
British journal: Clinical chemistry tests (i.e., h**ae**matocrit, h**ae**moglobin, and h**ae**maturia) were performed at a single study cent**re** to mini**mi**se variability between laboratories.	*In British English, "ae" for "e" in haem-containing words;* *"centre" rather than "center";* *"ise" rather than "ize" in verbs ending with "ize" (although British English increasingly accepts "ize", as long as it is used consistently).*
American research report: All histolo**gic** and histopathologic findings from the f**e**tuses confirmed the presence of multiple **e**demas.	*In American English, "al" omitted in adjectives such as "histological";* *"e" for "oe" in foetuses and "oedemas".*
European clinical study: This was a single-cent**re**, placebo-controlled study to determine the effects of the LH-RH analo**gue** on **oe**strogen levels in a p**ae**diatric population with central precocious puberty.	*European English = British English* *"centre" rather than "center";* *"analogue" rather than "analog";* *"oe" for "e" in "estrogen";* *"ae" for "e" in "pediatric".*
International textbook: The human brain is made up of billions of neurons. Each has a cell body, an axon, and many dendrites. The cell body contains a nucleus, which controls all of the cell's activities, and several other structures that perform specific functions. The axon, which is much, much narrower than the width of a human hair, extends out from the cell body and transmits messages to other neurons.	*International English = American English* *Text does not need any corrections.*

13.2 Solutions to Exercise 2

CORRECTED PUNCTUATION

1. Moreover, our findings are in good agreement with published data.
2. Medicinal materials which (or that) are produced from bovine sources are now being replaced by nonbovine materials.
3. CORRECT
4. The committee members concluded that the project is well structured and should go ahead as planned.
5. The trial participants were below 20 years of age and were able to read and understand the instructions.
6. We used a high-precision immunoassay.
7. All patients were followed up after the end of treatment.
8. The markedly improved manufacturing process resulted in a higher yield.
9. The company promises a 5-year shelf-life for the capsules.
10. This was a 5-month study, with the follow-up phase lasting 2 months.
11. Both a prospective and retrospective analysis were performed.
12. Although we have a competent staff, bottlenecks do occur.
13. The techniques used included TLC, HPLC, and NMR.
14. CORRECT, but do not use quotation marks when mentioning nausea next time in the text.
15. Is that book yours? Or better: Is this your book?
16. The new antihypertensive drug represents a genuine advance owing to its favorable pharmacokinetic profile.
17. The authors confirm that the data have not been published elsewhere (see authors' signatures).
18. The concentration of stabilizer in the medium was 0.5 mg/L (or $0.5 \text{ mg} \times \text{L}^{-1}$).
19. ACCEPTABLE, but the plural is preferred: The general practitioners are advised to refer their patients to an endocrinologist in such cases.
20. In our study, we used the novel imaging technique for the first time.
21. A deficiency of the trial was the limited number of plasma samples available for analysis. In fact, as many as 42% of samples were lost.
22. Scientific writers of a non-English origin may have to consult a good dictionary at times.
23. The in vitro findings agreed very well with the in vivo results.
24. The incidence of metabolic syndrome in the USA is estimated to be as high as 30% to 40%.
25. Delayed growth was common in this pediatric population (with growth hormone [GH] deficiency being the most frequent cause, in line with published literature [12, 13]).
26. ACCEPTABLE, but periods in suspensions may be omitted: Dr P. Smith and Mr A. Black were in charge.
27. CORRECT, but periods in academic titles may be omitted.
28. Our findings did not reveal any connection between the increased heart rate and duration of drug intake.

13.3 Solutions to Exercise 3

CORRECTED SENTENCES	COMMENTS
Fifteen patients were enrolled in the clinical study in Spain.	*Write out numbers at the beginning of a sentence. If the number is large, use a "bridging" term, e.g., "in total," or rearrange the sentence.*
A mean half-life of 2.5 h was calculated from the plasma concentrations of **8** male and **14** female rats.	*Numerals required for 8 and 14 because 14 exceeds 9, and because this is a series.*
After a further 4 h, we added H_2O (**5** mL) and NADH (**10** mL) to the incubation mixture.	*Numerals required for numbers in combination with units of measurement.*
The production campaign comprised lots of **5 kg**, **10 kg, and 20 kg** of raw material.	*Numerals required for numbers in combination with units of measurement.*
The patient was released from hospital after **5** months.	*Both the word "five" and the numeral are accepted but the numeral is preferred.*
After the left thoracotomy, dogs were allowed to recover for **3** days (or three days).	*Both the numeral and the word "three" are accepted but the numeral is preferred.*
Of the **71** patients taking part in this survey, only **20** attended all study visits. **A total of** 35 patients were lost to follow-up, and **15** patients withdrew prematurely from the study. **One** patient died.	*Numerals required in all cases because this is a series (except "one" because the number is at the beginning of the sentence).*
Overall, 11% of the cells had to be discarded.	*Numerals required in combination with the percentage mark.*
Intra-assay precision ranged from **89% to 99%**.	*Numerals required in combination with the percentage mark. Use "to" rather than a dash in texts.*

13.4 Solutions to Exercise 4

CORRECTED SENTENCES	COMMENTS
Table heading: Patient **D**ata of Efficacy and **T**olerability – a **S**ummary	*In titles, capitalize all "important" words (i.e., any word except articles, prepositions, and conjunctions).*
Alternatively: Patient data of efficacy and tolerability – a summary	*Alternatively, use normal sentence case if capitalization in titles is not used.*
Study title: Follow-**up S**tudy of X-**r**ay **F**indings in Patients **W**ho **H**ad Undergone **B**rain Surgery	*In titles, capitalize all "important" words. In "follow-up," "u" in the suffix "up" is not capitalized. In X-ray, "r" is not capitalized because of single-word meaning of the term.*
Alternatively: Follow-up study of X-ray findings in patients who had undergone brain surgery	*Alternatively, use normal sentence case if capitalization in titles is not used.*
Serious adverse events occurring in more than 10% of patients are listed in **T**able 2.	*Capitals in designations, e.g., Table 2. Better: Table 2 lists....*

(continued)

CORRECTED SENTENCES	COMMENTS
The new drug was tested in **W**istar rats, **c**ynomolgus monkeys, and **b**eagle **d**ogs.	*Capital "W" in Wistar (name). No capitals in "cynomolgus" and "beagle dogs" (generic terms).*
The boy had Asperger **a**utism in addition to his **a**ttention-deficit disorder.	*Capital "A" in "Asperger" correct (name). No capital in "autism" and "attention-deficit disorder" (generic nouns).*
In our study, **g**roup A was clearly more responsive than **g**roup B.	*"G" in "group" not capitalized (noncapitalized designator).*
Genetic analysis revealed an impairment of **c**hromosome 21.	*"C" in "chromosome" not capitalized (noncapitalized designator).*
Method 1 proved more reliable than method 2.	*"M" in "method" not capitalized (noncapitalized designator), except at the beginning of the sentence.*

13.5 Solutions to Exercise 5

CORRECTED SENTENCES	COMMENTS
Introduction: Jones et al. reported similar findings.	*Tense correct but sentence better in the active voice.*
Introduction: It has long been known that smoking **increases** the risk of cardiovascular disease.	*Present tense because established. (Note: 'it has long been known' is obsolete!)*
Methods: The method used for analysis of plasma concentrations of parent compound and metabolites was an HPLC technique with UV detection.	*Past tense because part of "Methods".*
Results: The epidemiological data collected in this clinical trial **are** listed in Table 1 of this report. *Or, better*: Table 1 of this report lists …	*Present tense because the table is part of the report. Make sentence active if possible.*
Results: The subclones containing the D-helix substitutions were reassembled into plasmid P.	*Past tense correct because part of "Results".*
Discussion: In our study; we **found** that there were significantly fewer CNS effects in mice receiving vehicle only than in those receiving the test compound. *Or, better*: In our study, there **were** significantly fewer CNS effects in mice receiving vehicle only than in those receiving the test compound.	*Past tense because reiteration of new findings.*
Discussion: Recently published work by Miller et al. [1] characterizes the chemical structure of this compound.	*Present tense correct because data are published.*

13.6 Solutions to Exercise 6

IMPROVED SENTENCES	COMMENTS
Thus, the rat proved an acceptable animal model to study the effects on the composition of colonic lipids and **the effects** mediated by colonic lipids.	*Parallelism restored by repeating "the effects".*
Under no circumstances was any subject **who had completed** the three treatments allowed to be randomized for a second course of treatment.	*Parallelism restored by removing the incorrect joining of "enrolled" and "completed." "Enrolled" deleted because any patient completing the study had enrolled in the study.*
The book, written for chemists and laboratory technicians, is expected to be most useful.	*Sentence is parallel – no change needed.*
In the subgroup analysis, there were no relevant differences in the frequency of adverse events **between men and women. Moreover, the frequencies of adverse events in the subpopulation and the complete population were similar**.	*Parallelism restored by separating the two prepositional phrases, using two independent sentences.*
Patients with stable disease or a complete or partial response and **patients for whom** no disease progression is documented may continue with the treatment until the planned study end.	*Parallelism restored by repeating the subject of the sentence ("patients").*
The American research group reported incidences that **were superior to those reported elsewhere** and were less variable than **earlier figures**.	*Parallelism restored by adding the missing object for "were superior" (i.e., "those reported elsewhere"). To avoid repetition of the term, "earlier figures" replaces "those reported elsewhere" in the second part of the sentence.*
The participating cardiologists reported that more than half of the diabetic patients suffering from hypertension were as easy to work with **as** other hypertensive patients. **They required no more time to treat and showed at least as good an improvement**.	*Parallelism restored by using two sentences and establishing the two comparators in the first sentence using the correct "as." No need to reiterate the comparators in the second sentence.*
When applying proper writing rules, you will save time **and** energy, **and you** will feel satisfied with your work.	*Parallelism of this compound sentence restored by adding the missing "and" and repeating the subject "you".*
The statistical method is described in 4.2, and the results **are** reported in 5.2.	*Parallelism restored by correcting the erroneously joined verb numbers (is/are).*

13.7 Solutions to Exercise 7

CORRECTED SENTENCES	COMMENTS
The database of this ACE inhibitor served as a model because this compound was the first member of the pharmacological class.	*The database is not the "first member" – it is the drug! Dangling participle ("being") removed by arranging syntax in a logical fashion.*
You can see a thin tissue lying on top of the gut.	*The sentence implies that you are lying on top of the gut. Participle ("lying") shifted to modify "tissue" rather than "you".*
While I (or the technician, chemist, pharmacist, etc.) was having lunch, the reaction mixture exploded.	*Did the reaction mixture have lunch? Adding the assumed subject restores parallelism.*
Statistical analysis of the data showed that *Salmonella* infections were indeed rare.	*Infections cannot analyze anything. Confusing participle ("analyzing") removed by making the sentence logical.*
The data indicate a large safety margin for the active drug because of the observed pharmacodynamic effect.	*Data do not "consider." Dangling participle ("considering") removed by rearranging syntax, placing emphasis on the data.*
After its introduction in 1968, trospium chloride was broadly used in patients with either gastrointestinal disorders or urinary dysfunction and was proven to be safe and efficacious.	*Confusing participle "introducing" modifies "it," i.e., trospium chloride, but poor syntax implies that "it" refers to "the broad clinical application." Sentence corrected by removing the dangling participle.*

13.8 Solutions to Exercise 8

CORRECTED SENTENCES	COMMENTS
Blood and urine samples were taken after 2 h and 4 h, respectively.	*"Respectively" used correctly if blood was taken after 2 h and urine after 4 h. If both blood and urine were taken at 2 h and 4 h, omit "respectively".*
At Visit 1, subjects received the necessary drug supply, a micturition diary to be filled in twice a day, and a full study description to be signed at the next visit.	*"Respectively" redundant because all items were given at the same time.*
Validation data obtained by the external laboratory showed good agreement with those generated in-house.	*"Respectively" redundant. Sentence corrected by rearranging syntax.*
The bulk supply and quantities needed for the Phase III studies were both produced by Product GmbH.	*"Respectively" redundant because both supplies were produced by the same manufacturer.*
The three referees commented on the poor quality of the figures, the confusing layout of some of the tables, and the incomplete description of the assay methods, respectively.	*"Respectively" used correctly if each of the three referees made one statement. If all referees commented on one or several deficiencies, omit "respectively".*
Values for t_{max} in rats, rabbits, and humans were 0.5 h, 1.4 h, and 3.8 h, respectively.	*"Respectively" used correctly.*

13.9 Solutions to Exercise 9

IMPROVED SENTENCES	COMMENTS
Treatment with a single tablet **is** as effective as a 7-day therapy with the cream [1].	*"Is" replaces the passive verb construction (has been shown). The sentence is not fully active, but the copula is preferable to the passive voice. The present tense is correct because the statement refers to a published finding.*
Usually, centrifugation for 15 min suffices to separate the two layers.	*The verb "suffices" is active.*
Immediately after the accident, the 80-year old woman was taken to the emergency department of the nearby hospital.	*Passive voice can be retained because the agent (i.e., the person taking the patient to hospital) is unknown and the action is clearly passive (i.e., the patient could not take herself to hospital).*
Miller et al. [2] **consider** direct DNA binding of the compound the most likely mechanism of mutagenic action.	*Active voice is appropriate because the agents (Miller et al.) are known. The present tense is correct because the statement refers to a published finding.*
We do not **share** the opinion held by Hunter et al.	*Use personal pronoun ("I" or "we") to make the sentence active.*
After noninvasive tests, biopsy **confirms** the diagnosis of a breast tumor.	*The active verb "confirms" shortens the sentence and clarifies the sequence of tests done.*
Subsequent magnetic resonance imaging supported our hypothesis.	*The verb "supported" is active.*
Test tubes used in clinical chemistry testing are made of glass.	*Passive voice is appropriate. Forcing the sentence into the active voice would render the message stilted and obscure.*
Two independent technicians **monitored** the behavior of the rats for 24 h.	*Active voice is appropriate because the agents (i.e., the technicians) are known.*
None of the comparators **proved** more potent in this experimental system.	*Active voice is appropriate because the agents (i.e., the comparators) are known.*
Table 3 **compares** our findings with literature data.	*Presentation of data, i.e., tables, figures, appendices, or other forms of displaying data, takes the active voice and present tense.*
Statistical analysis did not indicate any significant difference between the two treatments.	*The verb construction "did not indicate" is active.*

13.10 Solutions to Exercise 10

REPHRASED SENTENCES	CHANGE IN RATIO OF PREPOSITIONS TO OTHER WORDS
The following flowchart compares the qualitative methods **to** identify drugs **of** abuse.	*Before*: 6 prepositions, 18 words (*ratio 1/3*) *Now*: 2 prepositions, 12 words (*ratio 1/6*) *Active voice*
The following table shows the incidence **of** appetite suppression **in** American and Canadian school children receiving Ritalin.	*Before*: 10 prepositions, 30 words (*ratio 1/3*) *Now*: 2 prepositions, 17 words (*ratio approx. 1/8*) *Active voice*
We re-analyzed the data **from** mutation assays **to** study the underlying mechanism.	*Before*: 5 prepositions, 19 words (*ratio approx. 1/4*) *Now*: 2 prepositions, 12 words (*ratio 1/6*) *Active voice*

13.11 Solutions to Exercise 11

REPHRASED SENTENCES	NO. OF MODIFIERS
The responsible process change committee will review any proposals for changes to the validation process and equipment.	*Before*: 7 adjectives, 3 adverbs, 3 noun modifiers (*total 13 modifiers*) *Now*: 1 adjective, 3 noun modifiers (*total 4 modifiers*)
This statistically significant result contrasts with earlier reports documenting no drug effect.	*Before*: 6 adjectives, 3 adverbs, 1 noun modifier (*total 10 modifiers*) *Now*: 2 adjectives, 1 adverb, 1 noun modifier (*total 4 modifiers*)
We cannot explain the underlying mechanism without further technical analyses of this phenomenon.	*Before*: 4 adjectives, 5 adverbs (*total 9 modifiers*) *Now*: 3 adjectives (*total 3 modifiers*)

13.12 Solutions to Exercise 12

CORRECTED SENTENCES	COMMENTS
If a serious adverse event occurred, the study was terminated immediately.	*"Terminated immediately" implies that the study was terminated prematurely.*
The mice in the first experiment were heavier than those in the second experiment.	*"Heavier" can only be "in weight".*
For easy comparison, the results are plotted. Or: For easy comparison, the results are shown graphically.	*"Plotted graphically" says the same thing twice.*

(continued)

13.12 Solutions to Exercise 12

CORRECTED SENTENCES	COMMENTS
The staining was red.	*"Red" can only be "in color".*
The finding indicates a possible relationship between product stability and enzyme activity.	*Verbose terms such as "may potentially indicate" show the writer's uncertainty. "Indicate" is sufficient to express the justified assumption.*
Further work is needed to establish the facts.	*Facts are true by definition.*
Immune reaction occurred in all experiments.	*The unnecessary double negative renders the sentence long and confusing.*
We were astonished by the result.	*The end is the result, and the result is the end.*
The patient has no history of suicidal attempts.	*The history is the past, and suicide is invariably fatal.*
We believe that the hazards of this X-ray examination are minimal.	*"Extremely" is redundant because "minimal" already implies the least possible degree of hazard.*
The team reached a consensus before finalizing the protocol.	*"Consensus" means "to agree," which is the same as sharing an opinion.*
We selected the best clinical center for the study.	*"Unique" is the best. Would anyone be tempted to say the most best?*

References

Dictionaries

Dorland's illustrated medical dictionary. 32nd ed. Philadelphia: W.B. Saunders; 2011.
Merriam-Webster's collegiate dictionary. 11th ed. Springfield: Merriam-Webster Inc.; 2005.
New shorter Oxford English dictionary. Revised ed. USA: Oxford University Press; 1993.
USP dictionary of USAN and international drug names. United States Pharmacopeia; 2006. Available from http://www.uspusan.com/usan/license.html.
The Merck index. An encyclopedia of chemicals, drugs, and biologicals. 15th ed. Whitehouse Station: Merck & Co., Inc.; 2013.

Selected Books

Alley M. The craft of scientific writing, Corrected 3rd printing 1998. 3rd ed. New York: Springer; 2009.
Bonk RJ. Medical writing in drug development, A practical guide for pharmaceutical research. 3rd ed. New York: Haworth Press Inc.; 1998.
CBE manual for authors, editors, and publishers. Scientific style and format. The manual for authors, editors, and publishers. 6th ed. Cambridge: Cambridge University Press; 1994.
Davis M, Davis K, Dunagan M. Scientific papers and presentations. Effective scientific communication. 3rd ed. San Diego: Academic; 2012.
Day RA, Sakaduski N. Scientific English. A guide for scientists and other professionals. 3rd ed. Westport: Greenwood Publishing Group Inc.; 2011.
Day RA, Gastel B. How to write and publish a scientific paper. 7th ed. Westport: Greenwood Press; 2011.
Goodman NW, Edwards M, Martin B. Medical writing: a prescription for clarity. 3rd ed. Cambridge: Cambridge University Press; 2006.
Gowers E. Plain words. A guide to the use of English. His Majesty's Stationary Office; Reprint of Later 1948 edition; 1948.
Iverson C, Christiansen S, Flanagin A, et al. AMA manual of style: a guide for authors and editors. 10th ed. New York: Oxford University Press; 2007. Available from: http://www.amamanualofstyle.com.
Lippert H, Lehmann HP. SI units in medicine: an introduction to the international system of units with conversion tables and normal ranges. Baltimore: Urban and Schwarzenberg; 1978.
Matthews JR, Matthews RW. Successful scientific writing. A step-by-step guide for biological scientists. 2nd ed. Cambridge: Cambridge University Press; 2007.
Ribes R, Ros PR. Medical English. 1st ed. 2005. 2nd Printing 2008. Heidelberg: Springer; 2008.
Schwager E. Medical English usage and abusage. Phoenix: Oryx Press; 1991.
Swales JM. Writing scientific English. London: Thomas Nelson; 1971.

Taylor RB. Medical writing: a guide for clinicians, educators, and researchers. Heidelberg: Springer; 2011.

Truss L. Eats, shoots & leaves. The zero tolerance approach to punctuation. London: Harpercollins; 2009.

Published Literature

International Committee of Medical Journal Editors. Uniform requirements for manuscripts submitted to biomedical journals: writing and editing for biomedical publication. Available from: http://www.icmje.org.

The CONSORT statement. Available from: http://www.consort-statement.org. Updated Nov 2010.

The Lancet. Self-plagiarism: unintentional, harmless, or fraud? Lancet. 2009;374:664.

Vessal K, Habibzadeh F. Rules of the game of scientific writing: fair play and plagiarism. Lancet. 2007;369:6–41.

Wager E, Field EA, Grossman L. Good publication practice for pharmaceutical companies. Curr Med Res Opin. 2003;19(3):149–54. Available from: http://www.cmrojournal.com.

Printing and Binding: Stürtz GmbH, Würzburg